2009

HEALTH IS WEALTH

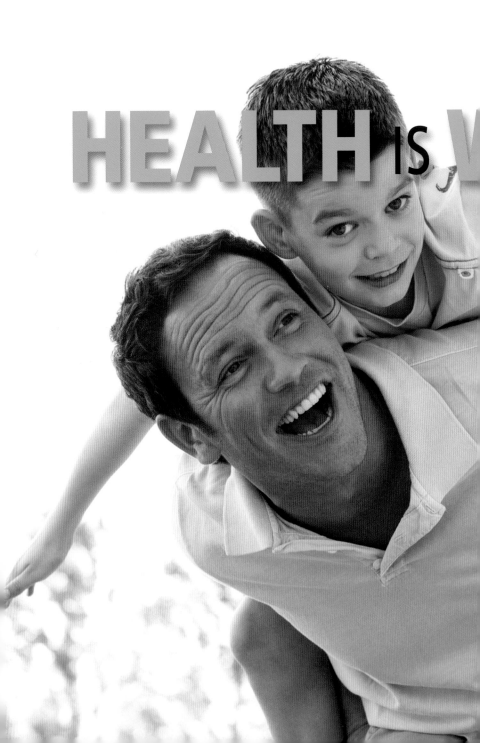

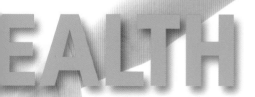

Ten Power Nutrients That Can Save You Money and Increase Your Odds of Living to Be 100

By
Louis Ignarro, Ph.D.
(1998 Nobel Laureate in Medicine
and author of *NO More Heart Disease*)

and
Andrew Myers, N.D.
(author of *Simple Health Value*)

Health Is Wealth
Ten Power Nutrients That Can Save You Money
and Increase Your Odds of Living to Be 100

by Louis Ignarro, Ph.D. and Andrew Myers, N.D.

Published by Health Value Publications

Cover Design by Cari Campbell Fuel3 Advertising
Interior Design by Nick Zelinger NZ Graphics

International Standard Book Number 13: 978 0 9790229-1-3

Printed in the United States of America

First Edition

Warning-Disclaimer

Health Value Publications and Drs. Ignarro and Myers have designed this book to provide information in regard to the subject matter covered. It is sold with the understanding that the publisher and author are not liable for the misconception or misuse of information provided. Every effort has been made to make this book as complete and accurate as possible. The purpose of this book is to educate. The authors and Health Value Publications shall have neither liability nor responsibility to any person or entity with respect to loss, damage or injury caused or alleged to be caused directly or indirectly by the information contained in this book. The information presented herein is in no way intended as a substitute for medical counseling.

It is recommended that you do not self diagnose. Proper medical care is critical to good health. If you have symptoms suggestive of an illness, please consult a physician—preferably a naturopath, holistic physician, or osteopath, chiropractor, or other natural health care specialist. If you are currently taking a prescription medication, you absolutely must consult your doctor before discontinuing it.

The Nobel Prize is a registered trademark of The Nobel Foundation. The image pictured on the cover of *Health Is Wealth* is Dr. Ignarro's actual prize awarded to him in 1998.

The Nobel Foundation has no affiliation with the authors in regards to this book and has not reviewed, approved or endorsed the content of *Health Is Wealth*.

For more information visit healthiswealth.net

From Dr. Louis Ignarro:

I dedicate this book to all who aspire to be healthy;
to those who have inspired me and to those who I can inspire.
Your healthy lifestyle is my success.

From Dr. Andrew Myers:

To Drew and Elke
Mom and Dad
and
Shannon
and
Amy
For all of their love and support.

Contents

"The doctor of the future will give no
medicine, but will interest her or his
patients in the care of the human frame,
in a proper diet, and in the cause
and prevention of disease."

– Thomas Edison

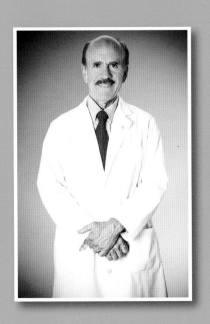

Introduction

YOU'VE BEEN BRAINWASHED. We're going to tell you the truth.

Along with the rest of us, you have been brought up to believe in a certain set of ideas about wellness and disease—a medical mythology—that our greater scientific understanding shows us is simply not true. These ideas have shaped how we live, how we maintain our health, how we deliver healthcare, and how we die. But, as we will reveal, those ideas are not only misguided but are also fundamentally false and harmful to your health, finances, and quality of life. Learning the truth can dramatically improve your well-being now— and decades from now—and may well give you added decades to enjoy living.

The medical mythology myths are:

1. Disease is inevitable as the human body ages, and we all inexorably progress from a state of health and vitality to one of disease and decrepitude.

2. Disease is a separate state than the state of being in health.

3. Once you have a disease, you are a fundamentally different being.

4. Once disease takes hold, it's just a matter of time before it "gets you."

5. The progression (or is it *regression*?) into more and more severe disease and disability is irreversible.

Do you find yourself accepting, often without thinking about them, that these ideas are true? If so, you're not alone. The late journalist Lynn Payer, author of the book *Disease Mongers: How Doctors, Drug Companies, and Insurers are Making You Feel Sick*, wrote that a confluence of some doctors, drug companies, patient advocacy groups, and the media combines to create fear (and thus a desire for treatment) around pseudo-diseases like "Chronic Fatigue" and "Restless Leg" Syndromes. Culture and communications influence, how we think about our bodies and our health as much as medical facts do.

How's this "disease-centric" approach working for us? It's hardly news that the developed world is experiencing a healthcare crisis. Families are being forced into bankruptcy due to skyrocketing healthcare costs for conditions for which they are not insured. Individuals are debilitated by conditions that are almost entirely preventable: cardiovascular disease, stroke, diabetes and more. What these disease processes have in common is that they are exacerbated, and in some cases caused by, habits that underlie the classic Western lifestyle: not getting enough exercise, enduring chronic psychological stress, eating too many high-fat, low-nutrient foods, drinking alcohol, and adopting unhealthy behaviors such as smoking. These habits nearly always lead to the development of obesity, cardiovascular disease, heart attack, stroke, cancer, or depression—the conditions that kill 70% of us. Thousands of studies and clinical research trials have shown us conclusively that 70% of deadly disease is due to lifestyle choices. As someone once said, "We have met the enemy and he is us."

So why did this knowledge not propel us toward improving our health? It didn't do so because we were bombarded with propaganda countermining our new knowledge, propaganda promoted by a $2.4 trillion medical-industrial-complex group, just as we were beginning to understand the root causes of disease. This group pays lip service to disease prevention, but its real message is that we should take no responsibility for our own health. Instead we should depend upon the next blockbuster drug to cure all our ailments. It's a disempowering message. Healthcare has degenerated into a situation where we wait to get sick, and then hope that a doctor will be able to fix the symptoms without ever having discovered or diagnosed the underlying problem or problems. But

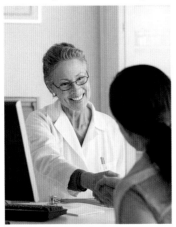

healthcare can, and should, be something far better: a collaboration among informed patients and physicians who are open to all aspects of conventional and complementary medicine. The fact is, *each of us is our own best doctor.*

A New Way Of Seeing Health

Our mission with *Health Is Wealth* is not to bash conventional medicine. Experts in natural and complementary medicine agree that when confronted with an acute problem, whether it is chest pain or a car accident, the best place to be is a technology-laden Western hospital. But when it comes to prevention of disease and the promotion of the underlying harmony of the human body, conventional healthcare leaves a lot to be desired. Its focus tends to be on treating symptoms after a person becomes ill. Any emphasis on nutrition, vitamin and mineral supplementation, exercise, meditation, or acupuncture is apt to be derided as "quackery," despite the proven benefits of each of these therapeutic approaches. "Disease-care" would actually be a more accurate name for the approach taken by the current system.

Our mission is to transform forever how you think about disease and health. By changing your perspective, you will change your choices, and better choices will lead to a thrilling enhancement of your wellness, energy, and longevity. What if we told you that you could avoid disease simply by promoting the optimal function of your body? What if we redefined disease? What if we told you that disease was not the inevitable end-point of our lives, but that, if properly supported, the body would continue to function optimally even at an advanced age? Would you believe us? Would you keep reading?

It's true. In these pages, we are going to present to you a fundamental redefinition of the concepts of disease and wellness. Listed below are the basic principles that *Health Is Wealth* is based upon:

1. *Disease* is just a word that conventional medicine has created to describe processes that are complex; processes that develop over a long period of time instead of in mere days or weeks.
2. Disease is not an unchanging state of being but a reversible and preventable process.
3. Disease is actually nothing more than a set of symptoms, which we will describe in detail, that your body exhibits to let you know it is deficient in certain key nutrients.
4. Vitality is the natural state of the human organism and can persist long into old age.

Let's discuss the word *disease*. Consider its literal meaning, "dis-ease:" a lack of ease. Its presence shows that your body is not experiencing the ease and comfort that it's supposed to experience—your body is falling short of its optimal level of wellness. When examining the concept of disease, taking into consideration its true definition, we are able to demonstrate that what we usually imagine to be an unnatural, organic process that devours us from

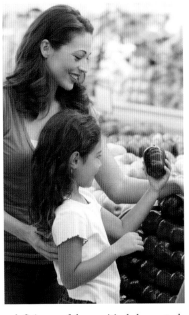

the inside—a malfunction of our biological machine—is actually a process that results from *deficiency*.

Instead of talking about disease, we should be talking about deficiencies that cause *dysfunction*. We say this because every human body requires a certain level of key elements—vitamins, minerals, amino acids, lipids, antioxidants and so forth—to function optimally. For each person, this level is unique, which is why healthcare needs to be customized for each person, rather than delivered in a standard fashion for a set of symptoms, with no consideration for the individual person. What we call *disease* is actually a state of *dysfunction* that occurs when a deficiency of these critical elements develops, over time, in a certain type of tissue. For example, when you deny the heart muscle the coenzyme Q10 for 40 years, cardiovascular disease is the result. The cardiovascular disease didn't strike suddenly; it slowly developed as the enzyme deficiency caused heart muscle degeneration.

The beautiful thing is that all it takes to reverse this process—to "cure" disease—is to provide the body with enough of the elements it needs to restore healthy function. The greater the damage, the more time it will take for proper levels of key nutrients—what we call the "Power Nutrients"—to restore optimal health, but it will happen. This is holistic, whole-person, long-view healthcare at its best: treating the underlying dysfunction, rather than prescribing a pill that just treats the symptoms.

The Link Between Health and Finance

If knowledge is power, then this should make you feel superhuman. This is a return to empowerment and a sense of control over how you feel, how you look, how you age, and even how long you live. It is the polar opposite of the "just take a pill" system. When you forget the word *disease* and focus on correcting deficiency, power over your health flows back into your own hands. Imagine a world based on the principles of *functional medicine*, in which the delivery of healthcare is personalized for each patient, doctor and patient work actively together as a team, and the crux of medical treatment is placed in preventing dysfunction by restoring and maintaining the optimal balance of all the body's systems.

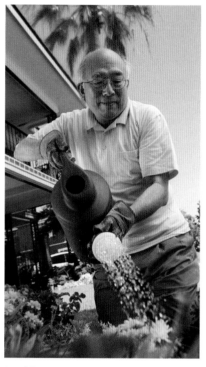

In this world, instead of careening from one health crisis to another as we age, we could take charge of our well-being and dramatically increase our odds of not getting sick in the first place. Of course, this isn't to say you will find a "New Age Fountain of Youth;" you're still going to age, experience some physical problems, and die one day, just like everyone else. But you can delay the onset of disability by decades and still be active and healthy when you're eighty or ninety, or even older, by rethinking what the term *disease* means and by choosing to empower yourself. In other words, a different world is possible, a world where our health, as our life progresses, is much more under our own control.

But changes like these will only come to pass if you reorient your thinking about disease, and that can only happen if you understand the connections between health and finance. We named this book *Health Is Wealth* for two reasons. Firstly, maintaining optimal health is one of the best ways to protect your financial well-being and increase your wealth over time. Secondly, the concepts behind successful financial investing are a perfect analogy to our ideas about disease and wellness. We will talk about this in more detail later in this book, but, basically, you should apply the same principles you use to build your wealth over the thirty or forty years of your working life, to maintaining your body's optimal health.

Health is like an investment account. When you are in a perfect state of vitality and getting all the Power Nutrients your tissues need to function at their best, your "health account" balance is at 100%, just what it should be. But when you suffer a deficiency of key nutrients, it's as if you're withdrawing money from that account. At first, the account has a lot of money in it, so small withdrawals don't make much difference. But over time, your balance starts to take real hits; eventually, you can't pay your bills. You start running a "vitality deficit," and your body reflects this by developing the problems we diagnose as disease. Only by putting "money" back into your account—only by restoring the balance of vital nutrients—can you return to health.

This incredible similarity between health and finance leads to two new terms that for us replace the outdated and vague terms "disease" and "health:"

> **BioDebt:** The state of nutritional deficiency that drains your wellness account.
>
> **BioWealth:** The state of nutritional abundance that leads to optimal function.

We will delve much more deeply into both these concepts, and into the connection between **BioWealth** and financial wealth, shortly. But to begin the discussion, we assert that it is well past time for us to begin applying the same disciplines to fostering maximal well-being that we apply to building a thriving retirement portfolio.

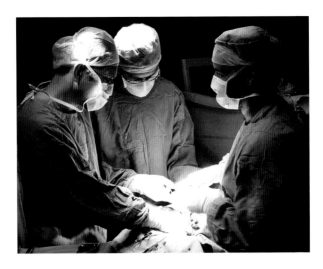

Who We Are

Dr. Louis Ignarro's scientific credentials are as good as they get. In 1998, he was awarded the Nobel Prize for Medicine, (along with Robert F. Furchgott and Ferid Murad), for his research discoveries showing the powerful ability of nitric oxide (or NO) to improve cardiovascular health and prevent heart disease. His groundbreaking work—the basis for his 2005 best-selling book, *NO More Heart Disease*—established Dr. Ignarro as perhaps the world's leading authority on the nutritional approach to cardiac wellness, along 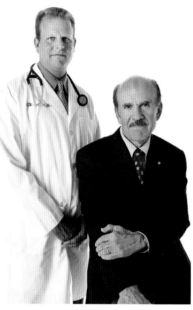 with making possible the development of Viagra. He holds a Ph.D. in pharmacology, is a distinguished professor of pharmacology at UCLA, and is a part-time professor at King Saud University in Riyadh, Saudi Arabia.

Dr. Ignarro has spent more than 30 years as a research scientist; seeking to understand the incredible role that nitric oxide plays in fostering optimal human health. One of his most important discoveries was that antioxidants, which reduce cell damage from free radicals, also increase nitric oxide levels by protecting blood vessel walls—which secrete nitric oxide—from damage. He has received countless awards in addition to his Nobel Prize, including the 2008 Distinguished Scientist Award from the American Heart Association and the 2007 Medal of Merit from the International Academy of Cardiovascular Sciences. He edits the journal *Nitric Oxide: Biology and Chemistry*, sits on numerous scientific advisory boards, and travels the world speaking to professional and lay audiences about the incredible power of nitric oxide.

While his research is personally rewarding and has great impact in the scientific world, Dr. Ignarro hopes, with the publication of *Health Is Wealth*, to reach and benefit a wider audience, an audience with whom he can share his knowledge of how the body functions from a biochemical standpoint and provide an educated understanding of the importance of good nutrition.

Dr. Andrew Myers, is a naturopathic physician whose career is based on a natural, food-centric, supplement-based approach to overall wellness and disease prevention through therapeutic lifestyle change. A speaker and advocate for the power of a natural, nutritional approach to improved health, he is also the author of *Simple Health Value*, a book about five easy changes people can make to improve their health. Drs. Ignarro and Myers are working together to define a new paradigm for the progression of degeneration in human bodies.

———

Health Is Wealth is a book based upon hard evidence, not one filled with pseudo-scientific speculation and overblown promises about so-called "wonder foods." Dr. Ignarro was as skeptical as most Western medical professionals are about the ability of food to function as medicine before he began to see for himself the incredibly beneficial effects of nitric oxide supportive supplements and foods on the vessels of the cardiovascular system. The old "If there's a disease, there's a drug for it…" philosophy was definitely the culture in which he was immersed. But as he observed the growing amount of empirical evidence proving the powerful effects of amino acids, antioxidants, and other key nutrients, he was forced to rethink his position. His is a rigorous, questing, scientific mind, and, when presented with overwhelming evidence of the ability of the 10 Power Nutrients to prevent and even reverse damage and dysfunction, he became convinced of their effectiveness.

This book is a synthesis of our combined 50 years' experience as a research scientist, and as a naturopathic physician, respectively. Our vision of health and disease prevention is based on our own clinical and laboratory experience combined with knowledge garnered from thousands of published research studies that we have synthesized into our unified theory of degenerative disease progression. Traditional research has a narrow field of vision; it looks at a single condition, a single nutrient, or a single drug. Very few studies have been designed to study simultaneously the effects of the many different nutrients that can influence our health. By doing our own meta-survey extraction from a massive body of current research, we have been able to examine nutrient interactions within the body's biochemical pathways and physiological functions. This work has uncovered vital relationships between specific nutrients and healthy tissues—relationships that demonstrate an unmistakable link between nutrient supplementation and **BioWealth**.

Strong scientific facts support every conclusion we make. As the healthcare crisis deepens, and support grows for the idea that our current "disease-care" system must be replaced with a new, different, better approach, we believe that we may be witnessing the beginning of the age of whole-body, whole-health medicine.

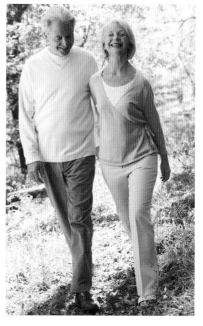

How *Health Is Wealth* Is Organized

Now that you know a little bit about us, let us introduce you to the flow of the remainder of our book. Our objectives with *Health Is Wealth* are to offer you a new definition of health and provide new insight into how disease should be viewed. We also want to provide you with specific information on how optimizing your health on a daily basis can provide significant financial benefits over the course of your life. As a means of grounding our recommendations within the health issues that many of us face, we decided to put our focus on the following three "health syndromes" which are familiar to all Americans:

1. Obesity, type 2 diabetes, and cardiovascular disease
2. Osteoarthritis and osteoporosis
3. Chronic stress, insomnia, and depression

We suspect you will wonder why we've chosen to group these conditions together into syndromes instead of dealing with them separately. We have two reasons, and understanding them will help you get more out of this book. First of all, many of the 10 key nutrients that we discuss are used in the same combinations to treat each of the conditions in the groupings of diseases that we have listed as one of our syndromes; reiterating the same treatment for each condition separately would be redundant. Secondly, and more importantly, the conditions we have listed together as a syndrome tend to cluster together, with one condition leading to another condition in the grouping. Obese individuals are far more likely than other people to develop type 2 diabetes, which in turn increases their risk of developing heart disease. Inactivity in older people can lead to arthritis, which generally causes people to be even more immobile, which can then result in the development of osteoporosis, especially in post-menopausal women.

If you look at these progressions as interconnected syndromes, you're far more likely to treat the root cause of the particular problem—a poor diet and lack of activity normally being the root cause of obesity, for instance—than to merely prescribe medication to suppress a specific symptom, such as being constantly out of breath, while ignoring the underlying heart disease, which often developed because of the obesity.

In *Health Is Wealth*, we want to teach you how to maximize your body's inherent wellness—your **BioWealth**—by "reverse engineering" the process of disease, in order to prevent dysfunction. Diseases and their associated and well-known symptoms—such as heart disease's chest pain, osteoporosis's brittle bones, depression's lethargy—are merely the end results of long and heretofore invisible processes that can be countermanded by nutrition. We're going to focus the bright spotlight of science on those processes to reveal to you their true nature.

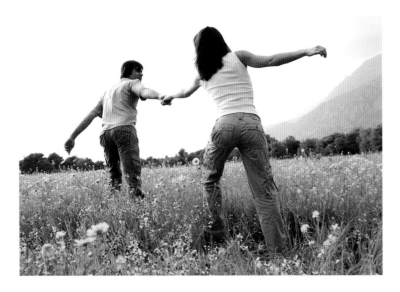

How to Use This Book

This book has what we consider to be a unique structure, one we hope will facilitate your getting the greatest possible insight from the material presented. Firstly, we discuss what it is that we call "disease," discussing what it really is. Then we go over, in great detail, the three syndromes we've listed above: obesity, type 2 diabetes, and cardiovascular disease; chronic stress, insomnia, and depression, and osteoarthritis and osteoporosis.

Following that, we have separate chapters for each of the 10 Power Nutrients that describe what the distinct nutrient is, what it does, where it can be found, and why it is important. In each of these chapters, we'll also list all the specific health conditions—the listed syndrome conditions and other conditions—that the nutrient is used for, and why it is that the nutrient is helpful for these conditions.

We have added eye-catching, informational sidebars to the book containing quick facts about the Power Nutrients, the health syndromes, and other fascinating aspects of wellness and natural medicine. You will also find that the pages of each Power Nutrient's chapter are all tabbed with an associated color. Whenever you find information about a nutrient in a sidebar, you can quickly find more information about that nutrient by using the matching color-coded pages to locate the nutrient's chapter. The signature Power Nutrient colors are as follows:

Alpha-Lipoic Acid

Amino Acids

Antioxidants

Chromium Picolinate

Coenzyme Q10

Essential Fatty Acids (EPA & DHA)

Glucosamine

Green Tea

Pomegranate

Vitamin D

We hope this system will help you get more from the book, and make it easy to find anything you are looking for.

Our website—www.healthiswealththebook.com—also offers additional information.

Our fervent intention is that this book will inspire you to take charge of your own health and longevity. We hope it will motivate you to set a goal for yourself to live to be a hundred years old, to live actively and proactively, and to make smart choices to prevent deficiency and degeneration in your body before it starts. For perhaps the first time in Western history, the choices and opportunities to do so are available to you. You have the power to remake the healthcare system for yourself and to become a full partner in your own wellness. We hope this book will be the first step—a gigantic first step—in a many-faceted process of developing the full strength of your own wellness, of taking back control of your body, and of living with all the vitality that is possible. If you take the initiative and do the work, you will change your life for the better, in ways you can hardly imagine now. We delight in the success you will have!

To your health,
Dr. Louis Ignarro
Dr. Andrew Myers

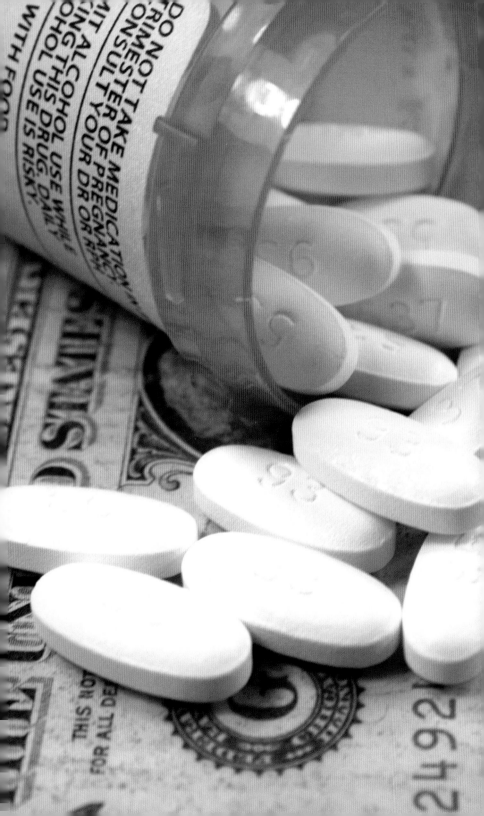

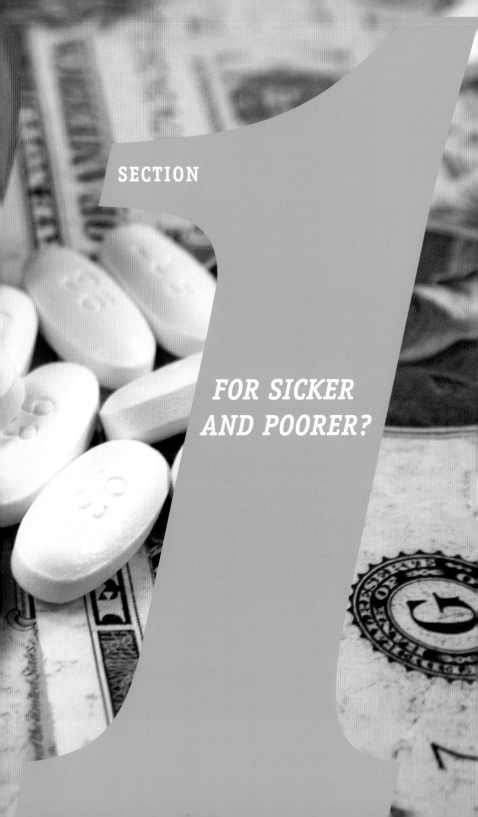

FOR SICKER
AND POORER?

Chapter One
Why Health Is Wealth

I got the bill for my surgery. Now I know what those doctors were wearing masks for.
—James H. Boren, politician and humorist

This is a book about wellness, so we're going to leave discussions of economic theory, foreclosures, and subprime loans to those with the qualifications to discuss them. But we can't ignore a simple, brutal, economic reality: it costs a lot when you get sick in this country. Health and wealth are intricately intertwined, and the strategies and mindsets that work for one also work for the other. That's why we've coined the terms "BioDebt" and "BioWealth," to replace the outdated terms "disease" and "health." If you approach taking care of your health with the same long-term thought and consideration you use when you are investing your money, you are likely to find yourself not only enjoying greater, lifelong vitality but also saving tens or even hundreds of thousands of dollars in money you won't have to spend on your health in the coming decades.

Every 30 seconds in the United States, someone files for bankruptcy, due in part to the enormous costs of treating a serious health problem without health insurance. Our economic meltdown, which eliminated millions of jobs and health benefits, has only exacerbated this problem.

The Cost of BioDebt

According to U.S. Census Bureau figures, the average cost of a hospital stay in the U.S. at the time the census was taken was more than $7,000. More recent figures from the National Coalition on Healthcare tell an even grimmer story:

- It cost $12,100 to provide health insurance coverage for a family of four in 2007.
- Healthcare spending in the U.S. is expected to reach $3 trillion a year by 2011, which is four times the amount spent on national defense.
- One in four Americans says his or her family has had a problem paying for medical care during the past year, which is up 7% over the past nine years. Nearly 30% say someone in their family has delayed medical care in the past year.
- A 2007 Harvard study showed that the average, out-of-pocket, medical debt for those who filed for bankruptcy was $12,000. The study noted that, contrary to common beliefs, 68% of those who filed for bankruptcy were covered by health insurance. The study also found that 50% of all bankruptcy filings were partly the result of unmanageable medical expenses.
- In early 2009, a report by the Department of Health and Human Services announced that, even as the economy was contracting and more people were losing health coverage, healthcare costs were rising to an unprecedented average of $8,160 per man, woman and child in the U.S.—and that costs were projected to rise to an average of $13,100 per person by 2018, accounting for a staggering 20% of all spending in our economy.
- As the recession cuts into tax receipts, Medicare's giant hospital trust fund is running out of cash more rapidly than projected, and could become insolvent as early as 2016—three years sooner than had been previously forecasted.

Not only can a chronic deficiency of essential Power Nutrients cause your body to fall away from its natural state of wellness and vitality, it can also wreak havoc with your financial stability. That's why we call it "BioDebt." Because serious financial difficulties ratchet up your level of chronic stress, you find yourself locked in a vicious cycle—sickness leads to financial duress, which results in greater stress, which brings about further dysfunction and degeneration—and so the cycle continues.

Chronic negative stress sends more people into BioDebt than any other factor. Stress, in and of itself, is not a negative thing; however, the physiological consequences of constantly engaging the body's "fight or flight" system are devastating to our wellness. "Eustress," a term coined by endocrinologist Hans Selye to describe the heart-pumping exhilaration that we feel under the pressure of a deadline, actually benefits us by increasing our ability to perform. Under the prompting of the sympathetic nervous system, the adrenal glands dump potent hormones into our bloodstream. Our minds race, our blood pressure increases, and we get a burst of giddy energy. There is nothing wrong with this type of stress, in small doses.

But the negative stress response evolved millennia ago to help us escape predators. It is designed to switch on for minutes and then shut down when the threat has passed, not to operate 24 hours a day, 7 days a week. But prompted by job worries, Wall Street woes, traffic, divided families, the Iraq war, and a thousand other crises, our "stress circuitry" seems frozen in the "ON" position. As Marnell Jameson wrote in the *Los Angeles Times*, reporting on the Stress in America study, "Chronic unresolved stress weakens the immune system, increasing our susceptibility to infections such as common colds and other viruses. And when stress increases, so does inflammation, contributing to stroke, arthritis, type 2 diabetes, periodontal disease and frailty. Additionally, studies have shown that the cumulative effects of unresolved psychological stress contribute to heart disease and high blood pressure."

Money doesn't just provide for tangible items such as food, clothing, shelter, retirement income, or stimulating the economy. Having money also affects well-being and longevity. In 2004, researchers from the Henry J. Kaiser Family Foundation found that increases in the cost of healthcare correlate to reductions in health insurance coverage. As the cost of insurance rises, fewer people carry coverage, and many of those who do buy lower-quality coverage that leaves them vulnerable to owing large percentages of the charges when expensive medical procedures or prescriptions are deemed necessary, or having to pay out a large amount of money before insurance coverage even begins each year. When people cannot afford health insurance at all, they stop seeing anyone for important optimizing measures—for care that isn't provoked by symptoms—such as regular physicals and cancer screenings. They stop getting any care that could expose medical situations before they become larger problems.

As we write this, public and private sector discussions about reforming healthcare are becoming more heated. Change would seem to be inevitable. But we have heard that healthcare is going to be reformed "soon" many times before. The system that delivers health-related services to millions of Americans is complex, entrenched, and profitable for corporate healthcare organizations and drug companies. Making any meaningful changes to it could take many years. Can we afford to wait for legislated reform, without knowing when it will come or what solution will result? For us, the answer is a resounding "No." It is time to reform our own health futures, and that reform begins by understanding the strong connection between wealth and health.

Wellness Is Like Investing

There's a reason why we came up with the term **BioWealth**, by which we mean living in a state of maximum vitality and energy that brings wealth to many different areas of life. First of all, in this state, you feel wonderfully well, both mentally and physically. You are able to engage fully in life and do the things you love instead of standing on the sideline because you "don't have the energy." Secondly, you are able to keep interventions by healthcare professionals to a minimum, thereby reducing your costs, reducing the impact on your time, and eliminating the stress that often comes with serious BioDebt. Imagine only seeing your personal physician once a year, for a regular, uneventful physical exam, and having a personal, collaborative consultation concerning all the things you're doing correctly to keep your body performing at its peak. Wouldn't that be a refreshing change?

When you get past the differing terminology and examine the objectives involved, you will find that personal wellness and personal finance are two sides of the same coin. For both of these, the ideal approach is to make small investments consistently over a long period of time in order to realize big gains after thirty or forty years.

Perhaps the best example of this is *compound interest*, which Albert Einstein called "the most powerful force in the universe." Putting away small amounts of money every month results in a very large sum of money, when compound interest is brought into the picture. If, at the age of 25 you begin to save $200 every month, and if you earn an average of 8% a year on these savings, by the time you are 65, you will have deposited only $96,000, but the value of what you have saved will be $705,872 before inflation. That's a substantial nest egg.

For another example, let's consider what happens when you walk regularly. Let's say that you take the train to work, but start getting off in the morning while it's still a mile away from the office, and walk the rest of the way in, and that you also walk a mile away from the office before boarding the train to go home. Working five days a week, you'll then be walking 10 miles each week—a mile getting to work and a mile getting back home. If you weigh 200 pounds when you start doing this, you will burn approximately 265 calories per day, or 1,325 calories a week, just from doing this much walking. You will lose one pound for every 3,500 calories burned, so if you keep to this walking schedule every work day for a year and don't increase the amount of calories you eat, you will lose approximately 19 pounds—just from walking five days a week. If your goal is to get down to a slender, fit 170 pounds, you can do it in 18 months by walking—with no other workout! Just as with investing, small measures taken consistently over the long term can result in incredible changes in your weight, fitness, and overall **BioWealth**.

When you focus on wellness and maintaining optimal function, instead of breakdown and degeneration, you are far more likely to make the same kind of investments in your health that you are hopefully making in your financial future. Doing so is financially logical. It makes good sense to spend 10 cents a day on supplemental vitamin C when you learn that doing so could prevent a heart attack in twenty years that could cost you $250,000. Not stopping dysfunction at the cellular level is basically the same thing as having debt that you're not paying down. It grows and accumulates, affecting you negatively. Eventually, when it reaches a critical level, things begin to fall apart and collections of cells start to exhibit distress. Biological "collection agents" call upon you, and your body goes into the physiological version of bankruptcy: breakdown and disability.

When you give your body a daily supply of the essential nutrients it needs to function at its peak level, you are investing in your present and future vitality. Doing this isn't always easy. It requires long-term vision, as does finance. Just as it takes discipline to consistently put money into the stock market month after month for years, resisting the temptation to cash out when the Dow plummets, it can seem like an act of faith to take antioxidants or coenzyme Q10 supplements every day for twenty years. But we can attest that it's not an act of *faith*; it's an act of *fact*. Well-supported scientific research results prove that when you consistently make "optimizing medicine" part of your personal care routine, you protect your vitality against future dysfunction. You are, to continue our financial comparison, making small, but daily, deposits into your **BioWealth** account. Over time, they really do add up.

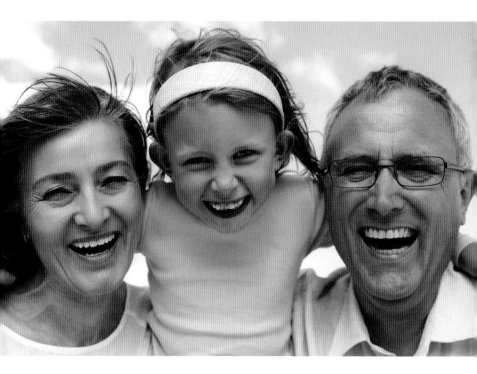

Rediscovering Responsibility

One of the consequences of our Western, drug-centric attitude toward our own bodies is that we are not proactive. We have ceded responsibility for our wellness to others. The prevailing public-health model, in the minds of health policy makers, physicians, medical educators, drug makers, and the general public, tends to be this:

a. Hope for the best and wait to get sick.

b. Go to a doctor and get drugs to manage symptoms.

c. Develop a chronic disease called "aging."

d. Suffer though increasing disability and receive intrusive treatment that does little to address the underlying causes of disease.

Clearly, something has to change. We can wait for our government to hand us new solutions on a silver platter, but that has not yet been a viable solution. The easiest and most effective factor to change is not our healthcare system, but our individual choices. No doctor or nurse, no matter how dedicated, will ever have the vested interest and concern for our well-being that we have. No one can force someone else to make sound decisions about his or her lifestyle; only individuals can do that. If we are to collectively re-engineer the landscape of health and healthcare in the United States and beyond, we must individually assume ultimate responsibility for the balance in our **BioWealth** accounts.

When you hire a financial advisor to manage your investments and steer you to a secure retirement, he or she may advise you about mutual funds or estate planning, but you are the one who makes the final financial decisions. Why should wellness be any different? We recommend that people begin to regard their physicians as medical advisors who provide expert medical advice and guidance. However, every individual must educate himself or herself in order to be able to make sound decisions that foster long-term optimal function of the body's systems, rather than just accepting short-term "Band-aid" solutions that make the symptoms "go away." Each of us has the power to become our own primary caregivers and to make decisions that will help stop potential health problems before they begin. By doing so, we will reduce our personal financial costs, lower the costs currently being passed on to our society, and transform our healthcare system into something that works for everyone.

The *Health Is Wealth* approach is to achieve health optimization by using supplemental nutrition to replenish vital elements that are constantly being depleted by our modern lifestyle. We will discuss this in much more detail later on in this book, but for now, we will summarize by saying that the combination of concentrated dosages of vital nutrients that you can deliver to your cells through supplementation, along with the fiber, phytonutrients, and energy provided to your body by eating healthful food, creates a powerful, wellness-promoting arsenal—one based on logic and backed by decades of proven scientific research.

A large subculture of individuals makes the choice to include things such as vegan or vegetarian diets, fitness, supplementation, or meditation as a part of their everyday lifestyle, but it's not a big enough group. We would love to see choices like these become a part of our mainstream culture, untainted by the label "alternative health," because they would bring about widespread improvements in vitality and decreases in disability and death from preventable conditions. But we aren't there yet. If the prospect of avoiding heart disease, diabetes, and cancer is not sufficient inducement to motivate a majority to adopt healthy behaviors, perhaps the idea of saving money in a challenging economy will.

> By feeding your body the right blend of key nutritional supplements, you will increase your odds of avoiding acute and chronic health conditions, reduce your healthcare costs, and, over your lifetime, save a small fortune.

Increasing the healthy choices you make will proportionally optimize both the condition of your body's health and the money you will save. It's common sense. If you maintain a normal weight, keep your stress level under control, keep your immune system tuned-up, eat a rich and varied diet, and give your body the key nutrients it needs through supplementation, you will, in turn, be less likely to get sick. You are also likely to find that any illness that does occur will be mild, require shorter hospital stays and fewer drugs, and be less likely to develop one of the "lifestyle killers:" heart attack, stroke, diabetes or cancer.

Also, it doesn't take a degree in economics to see that with healthcare and insurance costs already so incredibly expensive, and likely to increase by double-digits each year, true **BioWealth** can really save you a tremendous amount of money. You'll spend less on prescription medication, because you will fill fewer prescriptions. You'll get better rates, not only for health insurance, but also for life insurance. You'll need fewer visits to your primary care physician and fewer referrals to specialists. You'll spend less time in the hospital. You'll spend less time staying home from work because of illness, and you'll probably have more energy and be more productive. All of that, added together, equals less money spent, more money earned, and more cash left in your bank account.

But don't just take our word for it. Let's tally up some numbers and see how an ounce of prevention can deliver true financial benefits.

Health Is Wealth Benefit #1: Lower Healthcare Costs

According to the Centers for Disease Control and Prevention's (CDC) National Center for Health Statistics, the average American visits a doctor's office only three times a year. However, from 1996 to 2006, walk-in visits to doctor's offices, hospital outpatient clinics, and emergency rooms increased by 26%. To us, this suggests that a lack of preventive care is leading to a greater need for spontaneous, often urgent calls for care and a serious shortage of optimizing self-care.

In fact, according to the same data, only 19.2% of doctor visits were for optimizing care. We're letting health conditions go unchecked for longer and longer periods of time, and the result is that more serious illness develops. Hospital outpatient visits are up 43% for diabetes and 51% for high blood pressure. That was one reason given for why average out-of-pocket costs for deductibles, co-payments for medications, and co-insurance for physician and hospital visits rose 115%, from 2000 to 2005, per the *Health Care Expectations: Future Strategy and Direction* report from Hewitt Associates LLC.

Assuming that you have health insurance, how much do you pay as a copay when you see your doctor? Let's break it down for three situations: regular doctor visits, hospitalization, and heart bypass surgery:

Healthcare Costs Breakdown

Total Annual Dr. Visits (2 people)	Total Copays	Routine Tests (blood count & basic metabolic panel)	Optimizing Care Reduces Annual Visits To:	Annual savings
5	$38/visit, $190 total[1]	$85/visit, $425 total[2]	2	$179
Estimated hospitalizations in 20-year period, age 45-64	**Average total cost of 5-day stay**	**Out of pocket costs (deductible and 30% co-insurance)**	**Total cost (deductibles only) for 4 hospitalizations**	**20-year savings by cutting hospitalizations from 4 to 2 due to health optimization**
4	$19,400[3]	$6,820[4]	$27,280	$13,640
Heart bypass surgery	**Cost of bypass surgery**	**Average $1,000 deductible + your 30% co-insurance (assuming $15,000 max co-insurance payout**	**Cost of 10 years of brand name medications (statin, blood thinner, hypertension, anti-arrhythmia), 2 months of physical therapy, 2 month lost wages**	**Amount saved by avoiding the heart bypass**
22% of hospital surgeries for men[5]	$ 55,591[6]	$16,000	$70,660[6,7,8]	$86,660
Total amount saved through wellness optimization over 20 years:				**$103,880**

[1] U.S. Dept. of Health and Human Services
[2] *Focus*, May 2009
[3] Healthcare Cost and Utilization Project, February 2009
[4] Mercer 2008 U.S. National Health Plan Survey
[5] WebMD.com
[6] *Healthcare Blue Book*
[7] Blue Cross/Blue Shield of Tennessee
[8] U.S. Census Bureau

We're not figuring in factors like Medicare drug payments for older patients, because that would make the calculations too complex. But even if you take away the bypass, you would save about $17,000 over 20 years by simply avoiding extra doctor visits and hospitalizations. That's a year at a good state college for your oldest child or one heck of a family vacation!

Health Is Wealth Benefit #2: Lower Drug Costs

During a typical year, more than three billion prescriptions are written for Americans. Some of those are for short-term drugs for acute, temporary problems; drugs such as antibiotics or painkillers. But the most commonly prescribed drugs are those written for long-term treatment of chronic BioDebt conditions such as depression and high blood pressure. In fact, the three most commonly prescribed drugs in the U.S. are the antidepressants Prozac, Paxil, and Lexapro. Running a close second are blood pressure drugs such as Norvasc, Lopressor, and Lasix. Added all together, in 2004, seniors spent an average of $1,914 per year on prescription medication, according to a report from the Agency for Healthcare Research and Quality.

What if you could do away with all or most of, your prescription medications? How much would you save?

Drug Costs Breakdown				
Medications taken (brand names)	Annual cost (assuming 50% of drug costs covered by insurance)[1]	Optimizing care reduces medications to:	New annual cost (assuming 50% of drug costs covered by insurance)[1]	Annual savings
3: For cholesterol, hypertension, depression	$2,988	1: Beta blocker, lower dosage	$486	$2,502
Total 20-year savings on prescription drugs:				$50,040

[1] Blue Cross/Blue Shield of Tennessee

Health Is Wealth Benefit #3: Lower Insurance Costs

The cost of insurance seems to be rising as quickly as the quality and breadth of coverage are dropping. Even if you are lucky enough to be able to buy health insurance for yourself and your family through your employer, you don't escape the "bite." According to the Henry J. Kaiser Family Foundation, the average American worker paid about $3,300 per year for health insurance coverage in 2007—a 10% percent increase over 2006.

Becoming a healthy person by adopting an "optimization lifestyle" can help you reduce your insurance costs in two ways. First, if you have to find and buy private insurance through the open market, as many self-employed individuals do, you will normally get better rates if you control your weight, have normal blood pressure, and don't smoke. Secondly, if your fitness and overall health are so good that you can afford to take more risk than most, you can buy group insurance coverage with a higher deductible amount and larger copay share of costs. Since the amount of your deductible will usually only matter if you have a major hospitalization, you're essentially betting that you won't get a terrible disease—although you can't, of course, control accidents—so you won't ever have to pay the higher deductible. If you are comfortable with taking the risk because you've reduced the possibility of health problems occurring by taking proactive measures to be in the best health possible, you can reduce your premiums substantially.

Let's imagine that you're a corporate employee who has adopted a healthier lifestyle, and you are comfortable with doubling your deductible amount because you know that you've reduced your disease risk. Doing that reduces your annual contribution for your share of the payment for your company's insurance coverage.

Insurance Premium Breakdown		
Normal annual consumer share of company health insurance costs	Reduced cost after adoption of "optimization lifestyle" and higher deductible	Annual savings
$3,492[1]	$2,200	$1,292
Total 20-year savings on insurance premiums:		$25,840

[1] Kaiser Daily Health Policy Report, May 15, 2008

Health Is Wealth Benefit #4: Greater Productivity

Finally, how much income do you lose over the course of a year because you're too sick to work, if you are either paid on an hourly basis or you don't get any paid sick leave benefit from your employer? Disease, and resulting lost income because of it, is one of the major contributors to personal bankruptcy. For example, a study released in December 2008 showed that mental illness alone costs Americans at least $193 billion per year in lost earnings. When you add to that disability due to heart disease, respiratory diseases, diabetes, and other, often-preventable maladies, we would not be surprised if that total doubled to nearly $400 billion.

Divide $400 billion by 200 million (the approximate number of adults in the U.S.) and you get $2,000. It's likely that colds, flu, arthritis pain, or other problems cost you that much per year in lost wages. How much more would you earn if you enhanced your health and rarely, if ever, got sick, if you slept better, and if you handled work stress without wrecking your immune system?

Reduced Earnings Breakdown		
Typical annual earnings lost to illness	Annual earnings lost to illness after lifestyle optimization	Annual increase in income
$3,846[1]	$1,000	$2,846
Total 20-year savings through lifestyle optimization:		$56,920

[1] National Library of Medicine

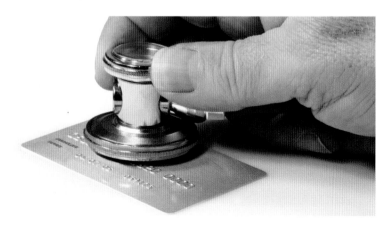

Health Is Wealth: The Bottom Line

So, given our hypothetical situations, how much more money might you have on hand to help you weather hard economic times if you used supplementation and other smart lifestyle choices to optimize your vitality to its peak level? Let's do the math.

Total *Health Is Wealth* Savings				
TYPE OF WEALTH DRAIN	ONE-YEAR SAVINGS	FIVE-YEAR SAVINGS	TEN-YEAR SAVINGS	TWENTY-YEAR SAVINGS
Doctor & Hospital Costs (not including bypass)	$850	$4,250	$8,500	$17,000
Drug Costs	$2,502	$12,510	$25,020	$50,040
Insurance Premiums	$1,292	$6,460	$12,920	$25,840
Lost Wages	$2,846	$14,230	$28,460	$56,920
Total	$7,490	$37,450	$74,900	$149,800

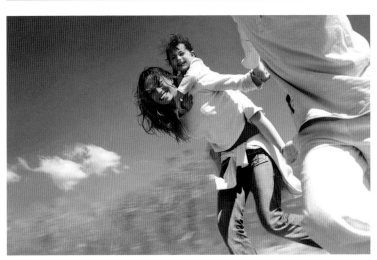

That's a lot of money, nearly $7,500 per year. Imagine you are investing that money for your retirement or putting it into a college education account, and that you earn 8% a year on it. Let's look at what you would have after 30 years from investing that money in the stock market (not accounting for inflation):

Year	Deposit	Balance
Year 1	$7,490	$7,490
Year 2	$7,490	$15,880
Year 3	$7,490	$24,967
Year 4	$7,490	$34,808
Year 5	$7,490	$45,466
Year 10	$7,490	$113,587
Year 15	$7,490	$215,076
Year 20	$7,490	$366,280
Year 25	$7,490	$591,551
Year 30	$7,490	$927,169

Just as with financial investing, the amount of money you can save by adopting an "optimization lifestyle" may not seem like much for a single year. But when you consider over a longer time period the possible costs you might have incurred, but instead have prevented, it is obviously a substantial amount. That much money can make an appreciable difference in peoples' lives.

Our approach offers so many potential gains, for such low risk, that it almost seems almost too good to be true. But if you begin and maintain proper supplementation, there's every likelihood that you will enjoy better overall health, more energy, lower stress, lower healthcare costs, higher work productivity, better quality of life, and more peace of mind—all without the side effects or cost of prescription drugs. That's because our nutritional strategy doesn't wait for dysfunction to occur and then try to repair the damage. It helps your body reach its full potential for wellness and prevents BioDebt from ever beginning.

Taking the nutritional route to health delivers benefits far beyond good health. *It returns control over your health to you, which is where it belongs.* Our health has really always been under our control, but most of us have been brainwashed into abdicating what should be our responsibility to doctors, hospitals, and drug companies. We don't think of our health as something that we can control. But no physician or drug can make us exercise, and they can't make us substitute brown rice and salmon for steak and mashed potatoes. They can't make us start taking amino acids and fiber and antioxidants. And they can't advise us about how to improve our financial fortunes by maximizing the performance of our incredible biological machines. We are in control of our finances in the same way we are in control of our wellness. That control gives us the power to create a promising future if we will just seize it.

Because the syndromes that ultimately disable and kill so many of us take decades of gradual breakdown and dysfunction to develop, it's our lifelong habits that will make the greatest difference in our wellness, vitality, and longevity. *We have the power to change everything, including our financial security, with our choices.*

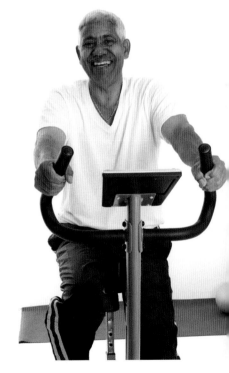

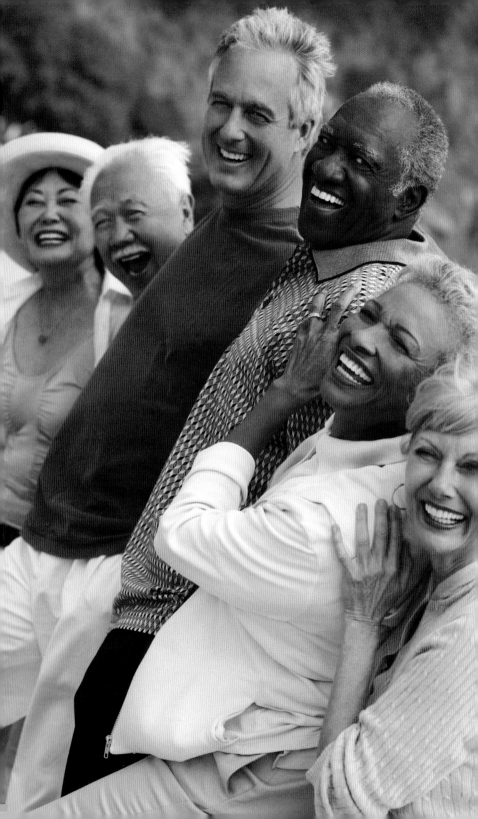

Chapter Two
Redefining Disease

The doctor is taught to be interested not in health but in disease. What the public is taught is that health is the cure for disease.

— *Ashley Montagu, anthropologist and humanist*

Residents of the island of Okinawa enjoy the highest average life expectancy of any group of people in the world: more than 81 years. Okinawa can lay claim to having the highest rate of people over age 100—34.7 centenarians per 100,000 residents—of any country in the world. Okinawans have the lowest rates of cancer and heart disease in the world. The Okinawa Centenarian Study has kept track of the elders of this society since the mid-1970s to learn why these particular people, in their 80s and even older, have clear arteries, fluid joints, strong sex drives, clear minds, and over-all excellent health.

From this study of Okinawans who have lived to an extremely old age and maintained a surprising amount of health and vigor throughout, the researchers learned that, while genetic advantages do exist, the main cause of the vitality observed lay in their lifestyle choices guided by traditional cultural patterns. Okinawans eat less than other people. They stop eating when they feel they are 80% full, a practice they call *Hara Hachi Bu*. Their high-fiber diet is rich in healthy fats and fruits, vegetables, fish, and soy foods such as tofu. They tend to hold deep spiritual beliefs and to be members of strong social circles that they belong to for decades.

These facts are crucial for our discussion in this chapter, because we are going to use them to help us drastically alter the way you look at the meaning of both health and disease. We're going to reveal the real, hidden mechanics of disease for the first time and show you how you can enjoy the same long-term vivacity that many Okinawans do. To begin, let's discuss what we mean when we use the word "disease."

The Meaning of Disease

Disease is an imprecise word that is used to describe a wide range of physical problems, ranging from cancer and influenza to depression and attention deficit disorder. But the intellectual and emotional connotations associated with the word are more dangerous than its lack of specificity. Disease is a negative term laden with a morbid sort of finality, as in, "I've got heart disease"; as in end of story. It equivocates illness to a prison sentence with no hope for appeal. This perception of disease has evolved from our conventional medical approach, which is often more focused on pronouncing a diagnosis or naming a disease than on the individual patient or the underlying physiological causes of the disease.

The concept of "disease" is poisonous to our long-term wellness because it is fatalistic. It encourages us to think of physical dysfunction as resembling being struck by lightning, it comes out of nowhere, it can't be protected against, and it's irreversible. Once you have a disease, there's nothing you can do about it. The best you can hope for is survival. This is the pervasive mentality in many societies. Disease simply arises. Once you have a disease, you have permanently changed. You're powerless to prevent its occurrence and powerless to alter it once it has appeared. That is the standard view of disease as modern Western medicine defines it. You have no control over your wellness and can only hope you will not develop debilitating physical breakdown.

The *Health Is Wealth* perspective of disease is completely different and is supported by a growing body of medical science. From this perspective, every human being, *in his or her natural state of being*, is a fully holistic entity operating with optimal functionality. In older medical traditions, it was believed that the body was self-regulating and that disease occurred only when self-regulation was disrupted. In contemporary terms, we call this condition a "feedback loop." Upon reaching maturity, the human body has everything it needs to maintain its peak function concerning organs, nerves, bones, muscles, and brain cells. It can handle the effects of moderate stress, cleanse toxins from its systems, and generally react as necessary to whatever occurs to it. It can perform these functions with incredible ease, provided it receives enough of the three key elements it requires: proper nutrition, proper exercise, and proper rest.

However, when this finely tuned system does not get the fuel, movement, and sleep it needs, its self-regulating feedback mechanisms become disrupted and imbalances and disharmony occur. When this happens, we call it "being sick."

> Starting from the position that your body's systems are designed to be in healthy alignment, ending sickness can be seen as merely a matter of bringing your systems back into dynamic alignment.

You're made to be well, not ill. *Health Is Wealth* does not focus on symptoms or on the endpoint of a health condition, but instead examines the processes that underlie the appearance of an illness; processes that begin to develop, and then progress, unchecked, over years or decades. Therefore, using the term "disease" to describe physiological afflictions is not explanatory or illustrative. These afflictions are actually dysfunctions of systems that can and will return to optimal function, once they are provided with what they need. Thus, cardiovascular disease is instead *cardiovascular dysfunction.* Type 2 diabetes is *blood sugar regulatory dysfunction.* Obesity is *metabolic dysfunction,* and so on. Our aim is not only to redefine what disease is, but also to explore the causes of our most serious conditions.

The use of this terminology is not merely different semantics. Words have power, and the way we think of physical dysfunction affects how empowered we feel we are to treat and prevent it, both as patients and clinicians. When we eliminate the word "disease" from our vocabulary and replace it with "dysfunction," we reveal the life-altering truth that disease, which we assume is unavoidable and irreversible, is actually *preventable* and *reversible.* Correct function can be restored. By preventing the dysfunction that leads to it, illness can be prevented.

As an example of this, medical science has insisted for decades that cardiovascular disease cannot be reversed and has insisted instead that prevention of further damage is all that can be done. But research such as Dr. Ignarro's Nobel-winning work on nitric oxide has proven that taking a supplement of the amino acid L-arginine can actually reverse cardiovascular dysfunction. Most of the common assumptions concerning what makes us ill and what we can do in response are simply wrong.

The Real Cause of Disease Revealed

Our bodies evolved to function optimally for many decades while being given a full spectrum of essential nutrients: vitamins, minerals, fatty acids, amino acids, and so on. Since many of us are now developing illnesses, it logically follows that something is robbing our bodies of those vital nutrients. That "something" is modern life.

- In 1988, the U.S. Surgeon General concluded that 15 out of 21 deaths involved nutritional deficiencies.
- There is a proliferation of nutrition-based research highlighting diseases linked to nutritional status.
- Research shows that taking 267 mg of Vitamin E daily reduces the risk of heart disease by 50%. But, on average, Westerners consume only 9.3 mg of Vitamin E each day.
- Research shows that taking 500 mg of Vitamin C daily can cut, premature death rates by 50% overall. But, on average, Westerners consume only 58 mg of Vitamin C each day.
- Research shows that taking omega-3 fatty acids helps prevent circulatory problems and reduces the incidence of stroke and heart disease. But, on average, Westerners consume only 150 mg of these vital lipids, which is less than 50% of the recommended intake.

Source: healthandgoodness.com

Before the Industrial Age began, our environment and lifestyle provided us with an abundance of the nutrients that our bodies require to remain healthy, to develop and maintain strong immune systems, and to function at peak performance. The majority of deaths in pre-industrial society resulted from accidents and infections. With our current, improved safety laws and sanitation handling, these causes of death have plummeted. Instead, we now die from lifestyle-related diseases that are nearly completely preventable: heart attacks, diabetes, strokes, and cancers. The underlying root cause of these and other diseases that kill us is a way of living that prevents us from getting enough of the nutrients we so desperately need, while at the same time putting more stress upon our bodies, which causes us to need even greater amounts of the nutrients than we originally did.

Here are some of the factors that are causing our "dysfunction epidemic:"

- Pollutants in our air and water (including cigarette smoke) damage cells and put our bodies in a constant state of emergency damage control.

- Toxins secreted by plastics, pesticides, and building materials cause a range of problems, from triggering asthma attacks to sparking tumor growth.

- Economic worries and a consumption-centric lifestyle lead to an environment in which our "fight or flight" adrenaline response is constantly switched on, flooding our bodies with powerful stress hormones that wreak havoc on everything from our blood vessel walls to our immune systems.

- Per the American Registry of Certified Professionals in Agronomy, Crops, and Soils, the mineral nutrient content of agricultural soils in the U.S. is becoming increasingly depleted. This means that even people who eat what should be a healthy diet are probably not getting enough of the minerals they need.

- We eat far too many processed foods that are rich in calories, fat, and sodium and far too few fruits, vegetables, fish, nuts, and seeds, and we fail to take nutritional supplements to offset the ill effects of our poor diet.

- We move too little and weigh too much. Per the Centers for Disease Control and Prevention, a full 66% of adult Americans are overweight or obese.

The irony here is that when we give our bodies the right amounts of essential nutrients, they are equipped to maintain normal function in the face of normal demands. But our high-stress, nutritionally-deficient, sedentary and sleep-deprived lifestyle and our toxic surroundings are unfortunately combining to *increase* the amount of vital nutrients that we need to take to keep the body's systems functioning normally. Taking the government's recommended daily dosage of core nutrients is no longer good enough.

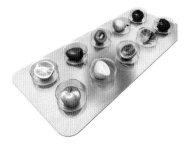

We call this negative circumstance *Nutrient Deficiency Syndrome*, or NDS. *This is the real cause of what we currently call disease.*

> Our unhealthful way of life is increasing our need for critical nutrients at precisely the time when our world is making it harder than it has ever been to obtain those nutrients.

The 3D Effect

We're not talking here about the effect you experience when sitting in a movie theatre wearing funny-looking, funny-colored glasses. The three Ds we are discussing are the three stages of Nutrient Deficiency Syndrome. These stages allow us to track NDS as it advances, until it becomes what we recognize as disease. Watching the progression of these stages shows us clearly that what we call disease is not a *state*, but instead is a *process*. During that process, the body, lacking the correct levels of some of the nutrients it desperately needs in order to function optimally, gradually breaks down at the cellular level. Eventually, seemingly out of nowhere, we display symptoms. Only then do we think, "I'm sick." But in reality, the process that led to those symptoms appearing almost certainly began years earlier.

These three Ds are the building blocks of Nutrient Deficiency Syndrome. The Ds we define here begin to occur when the body does not receive enough of the essential nutrients it needs. Unless the particular nutrients the body lacks are provided, one D will inevitably progress to the next. The three Ds are:

1. **Depletion**—Depletion occurs when the body's intake of one or more essential nutrients falls below the level that one or more of its systems need to function at its peak. An example of *depletion* is the body's level of coenzyme Q10, which is vital for heart muscle health, dropping below the level needed for total well being, due to dietary shortcomings and the demands of a stressful life.

2. **Deficiency**—Deficiency occurs when the chronic depletion of one or more essential nutrients begins to cause the breakdown of body systems at the cellular level. An example of *deficiency* appears when the heart muscle cells begin to show signs of damage after being deprived of sufficient levels of coenzyme Q10 for ten years.

3. **Dysfunction**—Dysfunction begins when such significant cellular damage has occurred that previously invisible harm begins to manifest as symptoms. An example of *dysfunction* is a person beginning to experience shortness of breath and chest pain, following an additional ten years of cellular breakdown due to deficiency.

Mainstream medicine would diagnosis this as *heart failure*, but our nutritional perspective defines it rather as *cardiovascular dysfunction*: the predictable end result of failing to provide necessary nutrition to the heart muscle over time.

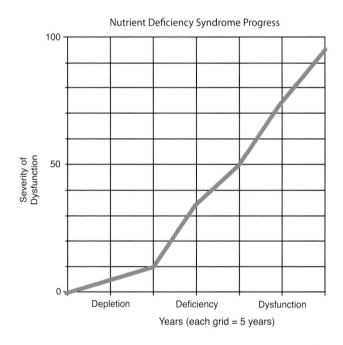

NDS is an accelerating process. When you enter a depletion stage, due to a lack of a certain nutrient, that state of depletion often contributes to the beginning of another. Your body is a holistic system. You could think of depleting it nutritionally as being comparable to an army pulling its left flank to attack an enemy, thereby forcing the right flank to cover the hole left in the line. When the right flank is stretched too thinly, the enemy is able to slip through the gap. In the same way, as a key nutrient is depleted, other systems are thrown out of balance. Your need for other nutrients grows; their levels become depleted, and the process compounds upon itself. The result is a vicious deficiency cycle—a domino effect—that increases damage at the cellular level. After enough time passes, you feel the symptoms of what you think is a new disease, but in reality, by the time you present with the symptoms of cardiovascular dysfunction or blood sugar regulatory dysfunction, your dysfunctional development has existed for decades.

Restorable, Reversible, Preventable

When you suffer clinical depression, your pain is not caused by a deficiency of Prozac™. You suffer because you lack vital neurochemicals that your body cannot produce, due to a deficiency of specific nutrients, and this deficiency prevents your brain from functioning optimally. This is why nutrition, rather than medication, is the key to reversing and preventing—in this case—mental dysfunction. Medication can't provide the essential vitamins, fatty acids, or antioxidants your body needs. It can only mask the symptoms caused by their lack.

The nature of Nutrient Depletion Syndrome means that there is real hope for restoring and maintaining optimal wellness and preventing serious health problems far into your old age. As with the Okinawans, maintaining your body at its peak level into your 70s, 80s, and beyond is a matter of returning your body to balance. You can interrupt the process of NDS at any point along its curve by re-introducing the vital nutrients that are currently at a deficient level in your body. Of course, the longer you wait to begin, and the greater your dysfunction, the more time it will take to repair the damage done and restore the

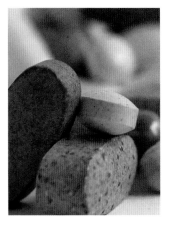

nutritional balance that will bring you back to optimal functionality. However, in time, by fulfilling your necessary nutritional "prescription," (and by adding, in proper measure, other important elements such as exercise and stress management), you can and will return to a state of true, good health.

Certainly, the best course of action is to prevent dysfunction altogether by choosing a diet that provides proper nutrition throughout your life. From the *Health Is*

Wealth perspective, that means including *nutritional supplementation* as part of your diet. Under ideal conditions, your cells receive the complete array of vital nutrients that keep your biological machine running at its optimal level. But we're no longer living a lifestyle that bestows ideal conditions. Instead our lives are complicated by conditions such as chronic stress, environmental pollution, and dietary poverty. Our cells now require *additional* essential nutrients to guard against damage, which leaves fewer nutrients available to do the work of maintaining normal, healthy function. As happens with any ecosystem, when available resources are spread too thinly, balance is lost and functions start to degrade.

We need a greater array of nutrients now—from coenzyme Q10 to fish oil to antioxidants—and it's virtually impossible to get them all, at sufficient levels, simply from the food that we eat. Food by itself cannot provide everything we need to maintain a healthy nutritional balance. But through a regimen of adding nutritional supplementation, it is possible to give your body's ecosystem what it needs to restore and maintain optimal energy, fitness, stamina, mental clarity, and immune system functionality. Supplementation is the key to preventing lethal dysfunctions from ever appearing in the first place. Planned supplementation is a good investment and one that will keep your biological "bank account" well-stocked.

BioDebt and BioWealth

This is why we invented the terms BioDebt and **BioWealth** as replacements for the outdated terms *disease* and *health*. Disease is a process that begins with depletion, with the body making withdrawal after withdrawal from a nutritional bank account that doesn't have enough deposits coming in. Eventually, the account becomes overdrawn and the penalties come in the form of symptoms: chest pain, joint pain, loss of energy, etc.

Proper nutrition via a balanced diet and supplementation supplies **BioWealth**, so that your cellular bank account is never overdrawn. There is a wealth of nutrients available to deal with the stresses of modern life, the changes caused by aging, and the needs of everyday function. Feeding these nutrients to your body means that depletion never occurs and you never progress to deficiency and dysfunction. **BioWealth** provides lifelong vitality and wellness. Proper nutrition is a renewable investment in your own stock that returns dividends to you in the form of greater vigor, more opportunity to enjoy life, more robust finances, and freedom from anxiety.

Cracking the Disease Code

Two possible futures lie before you and our entire society. We can stay the course with our current, fatalistic approach to health, viewing disease as something implacable and inevitable—the approach that is currently bankrupting us both personally and socially. Or we can embrace the holism of Nutrient Deficiency Syndrome and transform how we view disease, moving toward the concepts of BioDebt and **BioWealth** and taking responsibility for our future vitality and financial well-being. Let's see how those two scenarios are likely to play out for two typical Americans:

Patient A			
Age 44	Moderately Overweight	Sedentary	Poor Diet

Patient A chooses to take a passive approach to his well-being, based on several assumptions:

a. Disease is inevitable.
b. Staying healthy is a matter of luck.
c. If he gets sick, it's his doctor's job to "fix him."

At this point in his life, he is well into Nutrient Depletion Syndrome, though he is young enough that his longstanding nutritional deficiencies have not yet turned into symptoms. However, over the next 10 years, he begins to feel the signs of dysfunction, which he and his doctor dismiss as "just part of aging:" arthritis in his knees, pre-diabetes, obesity, and occasional cardiac arrhythmia.

By the time he's 60 years old, he has had both knees replaced, at a cost of $30,000. He takes seven prescription drugs daily and he can no longer engage in many of the activities he enjoyed as a younger man. He is taking more and more "sick days" due to illness and needing to be hospitalized, which reduces his income and increases the cost of his health insurance. Healthcare costs have also cut into his ability to save for his retirement, and the stress of worrying about his constant health problems has negatively impacted his wife's health.

Likely outcomes:

- Continuing health deterioration
- Financial impact: $300,000 in lost wages, healthcare costs, insurance premiums, and prescriptions
- Final years likely to be spent in infirmity
- Premature death

Patient B			
Age 42	Moderately Overweight	Sedentary	Average Diet

Patient B chooses to adopt the *Health Is Wealth* approach to her wellness from this point on, based on these scientifically-proven assumptions:

a. Disease is reversible and preventable.
b. Supplementation is the key to nutritional balance and **BioWealth**.
c. Her health is her responsibility.

She is well into Nutrient Depletion Syndrome, but gradually, as she begins to make new "deposits" into her nutritional bank account, she begins to restore optimal functionality. By age 47, a physical shows her arteries to be as clear as those of a healthy 30-year-old, she has the energy and vitality of someone 20 years younger, and she maintains a healthy weight and fitness level.

By age 60, she has sailed through menopause and shows no signs of the typical diseases of aging. Because of this, she spends nothing on prescription drugs, or extra doctor or hospital visits, giving her more money to spend on purchasing healthy organic foods and premium supplements. She intends to work until she is at least 70 years old, to increase her retirement fund. She is able to travel with her husband and to be as active as many people who are two decades younger than she.

Likely outcomes:

- Continuing **BioWealth** and vitality into her 80s and beyond
- Financial impact: $150,000 in additional savings due to low healthcare costs and continuing ability to work
- Great enjoyment of an active, vigorous lifestyle
- Life expectancy well beyond the average

Those hypothetical examples are not far from reality. Now that we have "cracked the code" of disease and identified what it really is, there is no reason any person should feel that his or her only option is to passively sit by and wait for deadly illness to strike. Redefining disease frees us from the prison sentence of inevitable physical decline.

In addition, as national single-payer health insurance slowly but surely reveals itself to be the natural structure for providing health insurance for our civilized society, and as the costs of traditional "disease-care" rise each year, even as millions suffer economic setbacks, our approach also presents the chance for greater freedom from financial strain. We have discussed some of the most direct and obvious ways that maintaining lifelong wellness can affect your wallet, but there are many others that are less obvious but have just as much impact. They include:

- Less emotional and mental strain from the stress of serious health problems, resulting in reduced or eliminated costs for counseling, anxiety drugs, etc.
- Reduced or eliminated costs for services needed to recover from illness, such as physical therapy and home care.
- Increased savings on the cost of life insurance.
- Less chance of needing costly long-term care at the end of life, which can cost as much as $70,000 annually.
- Increased energy and mental focus, leading to better job performance and higher earnings.
- Greater vitality and the ability to work longer and save more for retirement, leading to a more secure later life.

These are just a few of the other ways in which health equals wealth. The two are intimately connected, and a deficiency in one inevitably produces a deficiency in the other. Our financial well-being and our physical well-being are two parts of the same holistic system, and when we correct deficiencies in either, we improve both our current fortune and our future prospects for wellness and prosperity.

The Future

Redefining disease means understanding and accepting that each person has ultimate control over both whether he or she is likely to develop a serious physical dysfunction and over how long he or she will remain vital and healthy as time passes. Who wouldn't choose to be Patient B from the example above?

The key is the word *choose*. An understanding of Nutrient Deficiency Syndrome and of the real nature of disease shines a spotlight on an undeniable truth:

You, not your doctor or Big Pharma or the government, are the ultimate arbiter of how long and how well you will live, based on the choices you make.

You can choose to see this responsibility as either a frightening burden or an incredible opportunity to retake control of your wellness and vitality, returning to a balanced, holistic way of living. Remember that being well, whole, and vital is the way your body was designed to function. Wellness is your birthright. By learning what disease really is and how it comes to be, you have taken an important step toward eliminating it from your life.

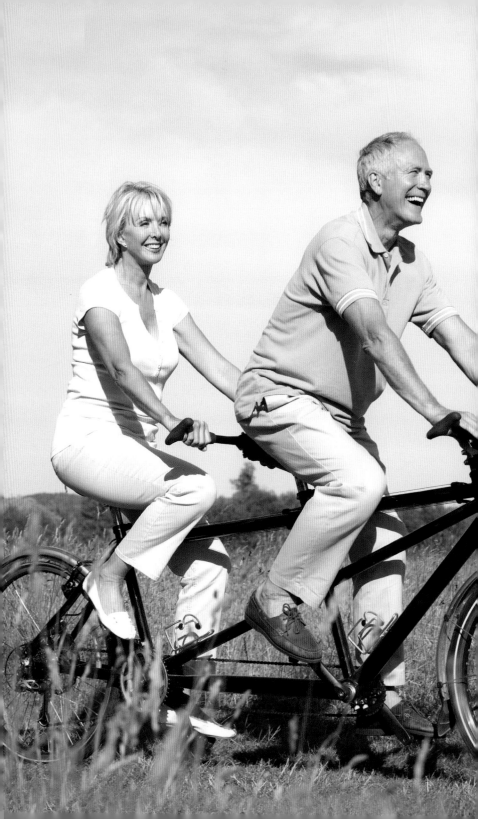

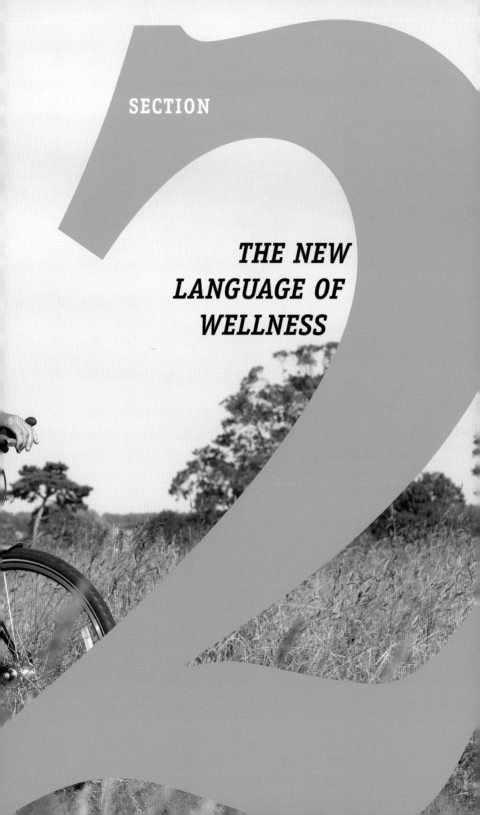

THE NEW LANGUAGE OF WELLNESS

Chapter Three
Symptoms and Syndromes

In putting our new understanding of disease and wellness to work to optimize our well-being, it's important that we have a clear lexicon—a definitive vocabulary—for discussing these powerful new concepts. Before we begin to talk about the surprising connection between common conditions, let's spend a few pages discussing some important facts about the nature of symptoms and syndromes.

First, here are some basic facts about symptoms and disease.

1. Disease is a constellation of symptoms that, when combined, are classified by conventional medicine as a "diagnosis." In conventional medicine, a diagnosis is tied to bureaucratic insurance reimbursement coding as much as it is to the disease process itself. Preventing symptoms from recurring becomes the focal point. This, understandably, focuses the attention of caregivers more on addressing these symptoms than on discerning and treating the underlying, systemic cause of the symptoms. Every symptom has a first principle that sets it in motion. When doctors try to merely erase symptoms (by prescribing anti-inflammatories for knee pain, for example), they are imitating gardeners who just prune branches while the roots of the tree wither and die.

2. Symptoms are signals that are our body's way of telling us what is wrong with its functionality—if we choose to listen. The value of symptoms lies in their ability to convey *information.* Severe joint pain does not equal osteoarthritis. It is rather a harbinger of the connective tissue dysfunction that is the root cause of arthritis, which could, in turn, be brought about by nutrient depletion, injury, obesity, or some combination of these.

Symptoms are one or two steps removed from the actual causes or dysfunctions that are associated with BioDebt. If we think in terms of layers, symptoms are superficial. They are the tip of the iceberg. The causative dysfunctions lie beneath the water line, deep within the essential mechanisms of our bodies. The question we must learn to ask when we experience a symptom is, "What underlying dysfunction is causing this and how can it be corrected?"

3. The personal history and biochemical individuality of each patient are critical but usually overlooked. No two people, even if they are manifesting the same symptoms, are exactly alike. Your dietary, exercise, behavioral, and genetic history is like no one else's. This must be taken into account when you and your healthcare professional work together to develop a treatment regimen to address the dysfunctions that are presenting as a spectrum of symptoms. "Off-the-rack" treatments may mask the basic symptoms, but without taking into account what a person eats, how he or she handles stress, and his or her job and physical/chemical environment, it is difficult, if not impossible, to properly treat core dysfunction.

4. Conventional physicians are trained to identify symptoms, and we, as patients, tend to do the same thing. Your doctor tells you that your blood pressure is high. You tell your spouse, "I have high blood pressure." You don't hear anyone, including physicians, say that you have "endothelial dysfunction due to obesity and a pro-inflammatory diet," even though this is the actual cause of your high blood pressure. Endothelial dysfunction is the root condition; high blood pressure is simply how it reveals itself.

The Functional Medicine Advantage

Conventional medicine is primarily concerned with intervening when dysfunctions break the surface and become visible or palpable symptoms such as pain, lesions, or organ failure. We label this "disease." Yet treating by masking symptoms does nothing more than keep disease at bay. Relieving foundational dysfunction requires more discernment and more time, but this ground-up approach has the potential to eliminate symptoms from the body.

Another vital way in which these two approaches differ is in the mechanisms they employ to treat conditions. Conventional medicine typically addresses conditions by manipulating the body from the outside. This is done via surgery, with drugs that inhibit or activate a certain biochemical reaction, or with toxic agents such as chemotherapy. In acute cases, these methods may be lifesaving, but this is partly because the conventional approach is, "Let's wait until it breaks, and then fix it."

In contrast, functional medicine works to bolster and optimize the body's natural functionality to correct dysfunctions. Let's use that high blood pressure example again. If you saw your doctor and your blood pressure reading was 160/100, he or she would put you on one or more medications that would treat your systolic/diastolic symptom—without ever correcting the core problem, which is a dysfunction in your endothelium. But a functional medicine specialist would recommend an approach designed to correct the dysfunction: exercise, a diet rich in whole, fresh plant foods, and a customized supplementation regimen which included taking the amino acid L-arginine.

There are several advantages to the functional medicine approach. First, rather than imposing change *upon* the body that causes unwanted side effects, it works *with* the body to restore harmony and utilize the body's natural ability to heal itself.

Secondly, conventional medicine is simply "done to" the patient. The underlying behaviors and choices that may contribute to heart disease or high blood pressure are often not addressed. But when a physician asks a patient to adopt new habits to restore healthy function, the patient has the opportunity to permanently alter unhealthy behaviors, reducing the risk that dysfunction and symptoms will return.

Third, conventional medicine pays little attention to the unique nature of 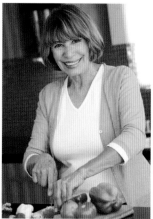 each patient. But with functional medicine, each treatment regimen is personal.

Finally, the functional approach is preventive and far more cost-effective. By working with patients to optimize their nutritional status early in life, functional medicine professionals can help patients avoid dysfunction and maintain long-term wellness.

Optimizing nutritional status can restore functionality and health balance after dysfunction has occurred, but it does take time for the body to reestablish normal biochemical and physiological processes.

The length of time needed to restore optimal function through supplementation and lifestyle improvement is difficult to predict and is, in many cases, correlated to the duration of the dysfunction. In other words, it's better to prevent than to cure. The *Health Is Wealth* approach excels at prevention.

What Is a Syndrome?

If you accumulate enough symptoms, you will have a syndrome. A syndrome is a cluster of biochemical and physiological dysfunctions that impact one or more systems in the body—such as the cardiovascular system, made up of the heart and blood vessels—and that shares common origins in terms of nutritional deficiency and poor lifestyle habits. All syndromes originate from the progress of the 3D Effect. What modern medicine calls "disease" is actually dysfunction brought on by the chronic, long-term nutritional deficiency we call Nutrient Deficiency Syndrome:

How the 3D Effect Becomes a Syndrome
Depletion ⇨ Deficiency ⇨ Dysfunction
Dysfunction = Symptom(s)
Multiple Concurrent, Interrelated Symptoms = Syndrome

Syndromes manifest as multiple dysfunctions that appear simultaneously in a patient as a result of the same deficiencies or lifestyle choices. The best known example may be the Metabolic Syndrome, a cluster of dysfunctions that exhibit symptoms including obesity around the waist, high blood pressure and high cholesterol, and that also predispose toward a higher risk of cardiovascular disease. The vital fact to understand is that these are not the diseases themselves. They are merely the symptoms that are the visible, measureable presentation of underlying dysfunction.

- High blood pressure is a *symptom* that can indicate many possible dysfunctions. One is located at the level of the endothelium, which is the thin layer of cells that line the blood vessels. In this dysfunction, the endothelial cells do not produce enough nitric oxide, which is a short-lived gas that promotes blood vessel relaxation. Chronic dehydration is another common dysfunction that presents with elevated blood pressure.

- Truncal obesity, the deposition of fat (adipose tissue) around the midsection, is a *symptom*. It is driven by a combination of dysfunctions that may include hormone imbalance, metabolic disruption, and insulin insensitivity.
- Elevated cholesterol is a *symptom* of a dysfunction of the liver and its ability to process fats and triglycerides.

Common Ground

The other critical factor to understand about syndromes is that they co-mingle and are progressive. Each is comprised of multiple individual dysfunctions that tend to occur together and they all stem from the same root nutritional cause and "co-escalate," meaning that as one dysfunction worsens, it makes the others worse as well.

- Obese individuals often develop type 2 diabetes.
- A majority of type 2 diabetics are obese.
- Type 2 diabetics often develop cardiovascular dysfunction that leads to heart failure.

Because the nutrient deficiencies that drive dysfunction are interactive, syndromes tend to have similar causes, rooted in Nutritional Deficiency Syndrome. Obese individuals share common deficiencies with type 2 diabetics and individuals with cardiovascular dysfunction. Patients experiencing osteoporosis will often exhibit the same lack of critical nutrients as those with osteoarthritis.

This interactivity carries an advantage as well. Because multiple aspects of a syndrome can stem from a deficiency of the same constellation of nutrients, restoring optimal levels of those nutrients can not only restore functionality in one area but can also relieve or even eliminate other symptoms within the syndrome. This is the essence of holistic medicine: treat a person as a unified system by using a unified nutritional, biochemical, kinetic, psychological, emotional, and behavioral perspective.

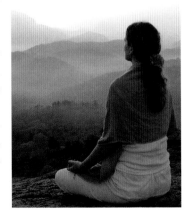

The Three Syndromes

We know that Nutrient Deficiency Syndrome (NDS) is the root cause of what is commonly called disease. Now we're going to examine three of the most common and dangerous syndromes from this fresh perspective. Based on the *Health Is Wealth* nutritional deficiency model, two major changes occur in our taxonomy—our classification—of disease:

1. Clusters of conditions such as high blood pressure and joint pain, which are commonly thought of as disorders to be treated, are demoted to symptoms that merely indicate a primary dysfunction.
2. The collections of symptoms commonly categorized by conventional medicine as diseases are identified instead as dysfunctions that make up but one aspect of the larger syndrome.

The syndrome can be thought of as a three-tiered pyramid:

SYNDROME
comprised
of multiple health
dysfunctions sharing
common nutritional causes

DYSFUNCTIONS
commonly viewed as separate "diseases"
but that actually manifest a deeper level of
dysfunction and share many common causal factors.

SYMPTOMS
such as chest pain, weakness or "the blues" that result from
long-term nutritional deficiency and that, when diagnosed together,
are classified by conventional medicine as "disease."

Nutrient Deficiency Syndrome and unhealthy lifestyle choices interconnect each level of the pyramid—from symptoms like high blood pressure or headaches to complex conditions like obesity or depression. What we have considered to be disparate diseases are actually components of one holistic dysfunction affecting the body at the cellular level.

The three critical syndromes we will discuss (and their component dysfunctions) are:

Sedentary-Inflammatory Syndrome, comprised of:
- Obesity (also called Metabolic Dysfunction)
- Type II Diabetes (also called Blood Sugar Regulatory Dysfunction)
- Cardiovascular Dysfunction (also called Endothelial Dysfunction)

Stress Imbalance Syndrome, comprised of:
- Stress
- Insomnia (also called Sleep Hormone Dysfunction)
- Depression (also called Neurochemical Dysfunction)

Bone Dysfunction Syndrome, comprised of:
- Osteoporosis (also called Bone Mineralization Dysfunction)
- Osteoarthritis (also called Connective Tissue Dysfunction)

In the upcoming chapters, we're going to mainly refer to these dysfunctional conditions by the names you're familiar with, for clarity's sake. But if you keep in mind the holistic approach, that at the heart of every symptom lies a system of the body out of biochemical balance, you will see that each syndrome is not an end in itself, but instead is the body's desperate attempt to draw attention to its dysfunction, so that through nutrition and lifestyle transformation, healing can occur and balance can be restored.

Chapter Four
Sedentary-Inflammatory Syndrome

(Obesity + Type 2 Diabetes + Cardiovascular Disease)

"Except for smoking, obesity is now the number one preventable cause of death in this country. 300,000 people die of obesity every year."

—*Dr. C. Everett Koop, former Surgeon General*

Obesity, type 2 diabetes, and cardiovascular dysfunction share a common set of symptoms (excess body fat, elevated blood sugar and insulin, insulin insensitivity, elevated cholesterol and triglycerides, endothelial dysfunction, and nitric oxide deficiency, to name a few) and nutrient deficiencies (in coenzyme Q10, L-arginine, chromium, Vitamin D, antioxidants and Omega-3 fatty acids). We could easily call it "Industrialized Lifestyle Syndrome" (and we considered that) because it's brought on by classic Western lifestyle choices: not getting enough exercise, eating too much high-fat fast and processed food, consuming too much red meat and saturated fat, eating too few fresh fruits, vegetables, nuts and seeds, and smoking.

What makes Sedentary-Inflammatory Syndrome so perilous is that one dysfunction predictably leads to another. According to 2002 findings by the International Obesity Task Force, 58% of type 2 diabetes cases can be attributed to a high Body Mass Index. Diabetes, in turn, increases the risk of cardiovascular dysfunction and heart failure, in great part because the combination of high cholesterol and uncontrolled blood sugar causes severe vascular inflammation that elevates the risk of blood clots, arterial blockage, and heart attack. Thus we arrive at "Sedentary-Inflammatory Syndrome."

Each separate dysfunction in Sedentary-Inflammatory Syndrome can be thought of as one "stage" on the path to the final and most severe dysfunction—in this case, heart disease that leads to heart attack, stroke, or heart failure. Once you begin experiencing the nutritional depletion that leads to obesity, unless you arrest its progress, you will develop symptoms like high cholesterol and insulin resistance that are also symptoms of type 2 diabetes. You could say that one bad turn leads to another.

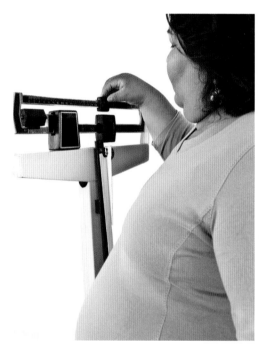

What Dysfunctions?

Each shortfall of a vital Power Nutrient produces its own spectrum of cellular dysfunctions. If we are to understand how these individual responses to nutritional depletion produce the macro-scale symptoms that we call disease, it's important to know which nutrient deficiencies produce which dysfunctions. What specific dysfunctions occur due to the deficiencies found in Sedentary-Inflammatory Syndrome?

Chromium
The chronic intake of sugar and refined starches leads to chromium depletion and chronically-elevated levels of insulin. Chromium deficiency impairs cellular insulin sensitivity and blood sugar metabolism.

Omega-3 Fatty Acids
Dietary intake of excess saturated fats paired with deficient intake of Omega-3 fatty acids (from fresh fish, fresh vegetables and whole grains) leads to pro-inflammatory conditions in the body. Inflammation promotes oxidation of cholesterol. Deficiency in Omega-3 fatty acids impairs the functionality of cell membranes and contributes to endothelial dysfunction.

Coenzyme Q10 (CoQ10)
Chronic depletion of CoQ10 and, in some people, negative drug interaction (statin drugs inhibit CoQ10 manufacture in the body) lead to reduced energy production in heart cells (mitochondrial dysfunction) and heart failure, impaired nitric oxide production (symptom – high blood pressure) and increased oxidation (free radical damage) in the cardiovascular system.

Vitamin D
Insufficient Vitamin D leads to increases in inflammation in the cardiovascular system and has been correlated with impaired blood sugar metabolism. Obesity is another cause of vitamin D deficiency, according to researchers, who found that even when dietary vitamin D intake and sun exposure are adequate, the vitamin becomes unavailable because it becomes lost when it is stored in a large amount of body fat.

Amino Acids
Insufficient levels of L-arginine lead to inadequate production of nitric oxide. When nitric oxide production is decreased, blood pressure increases, platelets become stickier (thickening blood), and oxidation in the cardiovascular system increases. Optimizing intake of L-citrulline helps the body to recycle L-arginine to form more nitric oxide. Insufficient intake of L-carnitine leads to reduced energy production in cells, including heart muscle cells (mitrochondrial dysfunction).

Antioxidants
Antioxidant deficiency leads to oxidative (free radical) damage to cholesterol, cells, and DNA throughout the cardiovascular system. Antioxidants extend the lifespan of nitric oxide, enhancing its activity throughout the cardiovascular system and beyond.

Supportive Nutrients
Green tea and pomegranate provide targeted antioxidant protection for important biochemical and physiological processes throughout the body, especially within the cardiovascular system.

Compensatory Depletion

Sedentary-Inflammatory Syndrome is also fertile ground for another extremely important concept: *compensatory depletion*. From a clinical perspective, obese people tend to be deficient in certain nutrients. This leads to *primary deficiencies*. But the choices that cause obesity frequently force the body to scavenge other vital nutrients to get the essential chemicals it needs to function. This then produces *compensatory* or *secondary* depletions of other strata key nutrients, which themselves can become deficiencies over time. These cascading depletions are the mechanism behind the progression from obesity to type 2 diabetes and then from diabetes to cardiovascular dysfunction. There is a class of supportive nutrients that can help to reduce the severity of these deficiencies. We can represent compensatory depletion this way:

Compensatory Depletion		
Primary Deficiency	**Secondary Depletion**	**Supportive Nutrients**
Chromium Picolinate	Amino Acids	Green Tea
Omega-3 Fatty Acids	Antioxidants	
CoQ10	Alpha Lipoic Acid	
Vitamin D		

The more nutrients you lack in the primary deficiency column, the easier it becomes for secondary nutrients to become so depleted that they slide over to the primary side. Compensatory depletion is like bad debt that breeds more debt. One shortfall in a set of key nutrients begets another. This leads to a deficiency that brings on a new dysfunction. This in turn breeds further nutritional depletion, deficiency, and dysfunction, until you have the equivalent of a boulder rolling downhill, picking up speed, and heading toward heart failure, disability and early death.

In the remainder of this chapter and the next two chapters concerning syndromes, we'll explore further the impact of compensatory depletion. You will see that proper nutrition, applied therapeutically and consistently, stops that boulder from beginning to roll. Let's begin by examining the three stages of Sedentary-Inflammatory Syndrome and how each feeds into the next.

Stage 1: Obesity (Metabolic Dysfunction)

Obesity is defined as a Body Mass Index (a ratio of weight to height) of 30 or higher. For many years, it was believed that heart disease was a result of the strain put on the heart by a severely overweight body, but that was simplistic. Next, cardiologists surmised that type 2 diabetes and high blood pressure, which are often results of obesity, were the mechanisms by which excess weight damaged the heart. But now we are discovering that the state of being obese, in and of itself, can lead to cardiovascular dysfunction and heart failure.

A study published in the *New England Journal of Medicine*, in 2002, showed that excess body weight increased the risk of heart failure, without even considering diabetes or hypertension as risk factors. Obesity can cause thickening of the wall of the heart's left ventricle—a condition called *left ventricular hypertrophy*—that can cause heart failure. Also, we now know that excess abdominal fat signals the liver to produce high levels of the "bad" cholesterol that can block arteries and provoke heart attack-causing blood clots.

There's also a 2004 study, performed in Australia, on 142 men and women of varying body weights who had no existing heart problems, high blood pressure, diabetes, or congestive heart failure. Researchers found that the hearts of the severely obese people had a dramatically reduced ability to pump blood, and refill with blood, during the period between heartbeats. The researchers also found a smaller but still significant dysfunction in the mildly obese volunteers. The likely cause: inflammation caused by metabolic changes.

Obesity causes prolonged inflammation of heart tissue and blood vessel walls and boosts heart failure risk. Some results from the Multiethnic Study of Atherosclerosis (hardening of the arteries) revealed that obese people are more likely to have higher levels of immune system proteins such as interleukin 6,

According to a study of healthy adults in Greece, adults who consumed more of the nutrients choline (by eating beef, potatoes, whole milk, fish, legumes, broccoli, eggs, and poultry) and betaine (by eating spinach, pasta, whole-wheat bread, and seafood) had lower levels of interleukin 6. Reduced blood pressure also appears to reduce this inflammation marker.

C-reactive protein and fibrinogen. At normal levels, these proteins are beneficial aspects of the immune system that cause inflammation to help wound healing. But at chronically high levels, they can cause serious damage to the cardiovascular system. In fact, doubling interleukin 6 levels alone increased heart failure risk by 84%.

"The biological effects of obesity on the heart are profound," said Dr. Joao Lima, professor of medicine and radiology at the Johns Hopkins School of Medicine. "Even if obese people feel otherwise healthy, there are measurable and early chemical signs of damage to their hearts, beyond the well-known implications for diabetes and high blood pressure."

To complete the picture, add the Metabolic Syndrome, which afflicts about 50 million Americans. As we said earlier, Metabolic Syndrome is typically diagnosed when a patient exhibits low "good" cholesterol, high "bad" cholesterol, high triglycerides, high blood pressure, and insulin resistance. Obesity can trigger every one of these conditions. The Metabolic Syndrome is the "perfect storm" of cardiovascular dysfunction risk because it can attack the heart and blood vessels from so many directions: coating arterial walls with sticky plaques, increasing inflammation that damages blood vessels, damaging the cardiovascular system by raising blood pressure, and causing abnormalities in the walls of the heart.

Insulin resistance, however, may be the greatest long-term concern with obesity. "Insulin resistance is probably one of the big mechanisms that causes people to get diabetes," says cardiologist Joseph Johns. "We've learned now that in people that have too many fat cells…those fat cells are releasing a lot of chemicals that make the body resistant to the effects of insulin. Particularly, it makes the muscle resistant to the effects of insulin so it makes the body pump

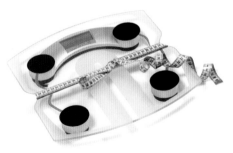

out more and more insulin for the blood sugar to be taken out of the muscle. Eventually the pancreas burns out and people get diabetes. Insulin resistance is the underlying reason we have Metabolic Syndrome."

Obesity also begins the downward slide of compensatory depletion of Power Nutrients. We've spent a lot of time on obesity, but it's worth the ink. It's the single most serious BioDebt source facing Western culture. Obese people tend to exhibit the following deficiencies and depletions:

Compensatory Depletion: Obesity		
Primary Deficiency	**Secondary Depletion**	**Supportive Nutrients**
Chromium Picolinate	Amino Acids	Green Tea
Omega-3 Fatty Acids	Antioxidants	
CoQ10	Alpha Lipoic Acid	
Vitamin D		

Stage 2: Type 2 Diabetes (Blood Sugar Regulatory Dysfunction)

Type 1 diabetes is caused by a genetic abnormality that prevents the pancreas from producing enough insulin. It has nothing to do with lifestyle. Type 2 diabetes, however, is caused by the gradual development of insulin resistance that eventually "burns out" the pancreas' ability to produce enough insulin to regulate the body's blood glucose levels. Type 2 diabetes can afflict people who are not overweight or obese, but it is strongly linked to high Body Mass Index, sedentary lifestyle, and the insulin resistance that often results.

Type 2 diabetes has become an epidemic, due in great part to the rapid increase in overweight and obesity in the U.S. According to government data released in October 2008, the rate of new diabetes cases in the U.S. has nearly doubled in the last 10 years, with 90% of them the type 2 diabetes variant. In fact, according to the Centers for Disease Control and Prevention, approximately 8% of Americans (about 24 million people) have the disease. Another 57 million are thought to have the blood sugar abnormalities known as "pre-diabetes," putting them at risk for developing the full-blown disease. Perhaps most disturbing of all, the rate of type 2 diabetes development in children is on the rise because of a jump in the rate of childhood obesity. Diabetes has become a lifestyle, evidenced by the fact that many major retailers have entire sections of their stores dedicated to diabetes books, magazines, foods, and care products.

Diabetes is the seventh-leading cause of death in the country. The main cause of death for diabetics is cardiovascular dysfunction. People with diabetes can also suffer from kidney failure, blindness, and circulatory problems leading to amputations. In addition, a person with diabetes has a 200% to 400% greater risk of dying from a heart attack or stroke than someone does who is not obese and who has already survived a heart attack. Diabetes contributes to the progression of Sedentary-Inflammatory Syndrome in other ways as well:

- By affecting the "master switches" that determine the body's levels of fats, lipids, and glucose, and by causing more plaques to be deposited on arterial walls.

- By stressing and damaging the endothelium—the artery wall that produces nitric oxide, which is the chemical that dilates blood vessels and allows them to relax, thereby lowering blood pressure and reducing the load on the heart.

Type 2 diabetes is so detrimental to cardiovascular function that, in a 2005 study at the Bloomberg School of Public Health's Department of Epidemiology, researchers found that each *1% increase* in a type of hemoglobin associated with long-term high glucose levels correlated to a *14% increase in heart disease risk.* The link between diabetes and cardiovascular dysfunction is no coincidence.

Type 2 diabetes continues the compensatory depletion slide as more nutrients become chronically depleted. Diabetics commonly exhibit the following deficiencies and depletions:

Compensatory Depletion: Diabetes (Type 2)		
Primary Deficiency	**Secondary Depletion**	**Supportive Nutrients**
Chromium Picolinate Omega-3 Fatty Acids CoQ10 Vitamin D Amino Acids Antioxidants (Alpha Lipoic Acid included)	⬅	Green Tea Pomegranate

Note that the previously depleted nutrients, Vitamin D, amino acids and antioxidants, have migrated to the Primary Deficiency column. This is because by the time the patient's condition has progressed to type 2 Diabetes, previously depleted nutrients have reached such low levels that they have begun to cause chronic dysfunctions, and are thus classified as deficient.

Stage 3: Cardiovascular Dysfunction (Endothelial Dysfunction)

We call cardiovascular dysfunction (CVD) "Endothelial Dysfunction" because it can be legitimately viewed as a problem with the *endothelium*: the lining of the blood vessels. Over time, obesity and diabetes lead to high cholesterol and triglyceride levels, high blood sugar, and high blood pressure. These conditions damage the endothelium, clog it with plaque deposits, and cause chronic inflammation. Those situations in turn trigger the vascular blockage, heart muscle damage, and obstructed blood flow we call cardiovascular disease. They also lead to blood clots, stroke, cardiac arrhythmia, heart failure, and heart attack.

CVD is the number-one killer of Americans. According to the American Heart Association (AHA), in 2008 an estimated 770,000 Americans had some type of new coronary attack and approximately 430,000 had a repeat cardiac episode, ranging from chest pain to a full-blown heart attack. The AHA estimates that an American has a cardiac event every 26 seconds and that every minute someone dies from one.

While it is true, according to the AHA, that deaths from CVD declined by 24.7% from 1994 to 2004, one out of every 2.8 deaths in the U.S. is still due to CVD. Since this is a condition that is overwhelmingly the product of lifestyle choices, that's an unacceptable rate. It's as if 500,000 people a year were voluntarily subjecting themselves to unwarranted suffering, choosing obesity, a low-nutrient, high simple carbohydrate diet, and a sedentary lifestyle. We now know that even small increases in blood sugar can be red flags for increased cholesterol levels and arterial blockage.

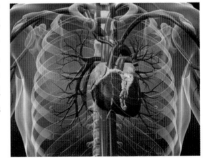

"Average Joe America goes to his doctor and hears he has borderline high blood pressure, his bad cholesterol is a little high, his good cholesterol is a little low, his blood sugar is getting up there—no red flags, just borderline," says Laurence S. Sperling, MD, director of the Emory Heart Center risk reduction program in WebMD.com. "But now we know that being borderline carries a significant risk. Doctors have to recommend realistic lifestyle changes and consider medications to lower these risks."

Just as worrisome is the increase in hypertension or high blood pressure, one of the major risk factors for cardiovascular dysfunction and stroke and the most commonly diagnosed condition in the U.S. With increased body weight and the artery damaging effects of diabetes, high blood pressure is on the rise. According to an American Heart Association panel, so is the prevalence of drug-resistant hypertension.

The drugs that bring down high blood pressure have not stopped working. But the people who are being treated for the condition are becoming sicker, per a 2008 report in the journal *Hypertension*. Many have diabetes due to obesity, and the kidney damage that type 2 diabetes causes can make it difficult for the body to eliminate excess fluids, leading to stubbornly high blood pressure that further damages the kidneys—a vicious cycle.

If you have diabetes and are carrying around 50, 75 or 100 pounds of extra weight, you're going to have multiple health problems that mutually reinforce and worsen each other, elevating to frightening levels your risk of a life-threatening CVD. Cardiovascular dysfunction also completes the devastating depletion of vital nutrients so necessary for cardiovascular health. People with CVD tend to exhibit the same deficiencies and depletions as type 2 diabetics, further solidifying the link between the two conditions.

Compensatory Depletion: Cardiovascular Disease		
Primary Deficiency	**Secondary Depletion**	**Supportive Nutrients**
Chromium Picolinate Omega-3 Fatty Acids CoQ10 Vitamin D Amino Acids Antioxidants (Alpha Lipoic Acid included)	⬅	Green Tea Pomegranate

Preventing Sedentary-Inflammatory Syndrome

There is no magic bullet for Sedentary-Inflammatory Syndrome. Reducing weight is the most important step. Numerous studies have shown that even moderate reductions in body weight can produce significant drops in blood pressure, cholesterol level, and blood sugar. The goals for reversing or preventing Sedentary-Inflammatory Syndrome are:

- Reduce body weight
- Increase physical activity
- Reduce LDL cholesterol levels
- Reduce fasting glucose levels
- Reduce blood pressure

Contrary to common medical belief, long-term replenishment of the body's stores of vital nutrients—repaying the body's **BioWealth**—can reverse much of the damage caused by inflammation, hypertension, and poor nutrition, reversing the symptoms and disability brought about by Sedentary-Inflammatory Syndrome. From a nutrient depletion perspective, the two main steps you can take are to improve your diet and to add Power Nutrient supplementation to your daily routine.

Dietary Changes
Eat more fresh fruits and vegetables.
Cut down on processed and fast food.
Replace simple carbohydrates like white bread and sugar with complex carbohydrates like brown rice and whole grains.
Replace red meat with fish, especially oily, cold-water fish.
Eat more healthy fats like avocado, nuts, and olive oil.
Practice portion control. The average adult needs no more than 2500 calories per day.
Eat 5-6 small meals throughout the day to keep your metabolism going and burning more calories.
Drink at least 64 ounces of water daily. It helps you feel full.

Power Nutrient supplements
Coenzyme Q10 (CoQ10) supports heart health and lowers blood pressure.
Amino Acids—The amino acids L-arginine and L-citrulline increase production of nitric oxide, the key chemical that relaxes blood vessels.
Antioxidants—Vitamin E has shown the ability to reduce the oxidation of bad LDL cholesterol, while Vitamin C has been shown to reduce production of it altogether. Antioxidants also make nitric oxide more effective at increasing blood flow.
Chromium Picolinate —This trace mineral has proven effective in regulating blood sugar levels.
Omega-3 Fatty Acids—The omega-3 fatty acids EPA and DHA have been shown to regulate cardiac rhythm, reduce the risk of arrhythmias, lower triglyceride levels, reduce arterial plaques, and lower blood pressure.
Vitamin D—This vitamin reduces the risk of cardiac death.
Green Tea—This tea delivers antioxidants, amino acids, and important phytochemicals in one package.
Pomegranate—Rich in antioxidants, pomegranate protects nitric oxide and promotes cardiovascular function.

What It Can Cost

As we have already seen, the financial impact of BioDebt can be staggering, and nothing carries with it a more potentially ruinous cost than the collection of dysfunctions behind Sedentary-Inflammatory Syndrome. When you consider the total possible expenses involved in treating and managing the consequences of obesity, type 2 diabetes and CVD, it's clear that taking small, relatively inexpensive steps to prevent or reverse these cascading conditions can not only lengthen and improve life, but can increase the odds of having enough money to enjoy those extra years.

Hypothetical Total Costs of Managing Sedentary-Inflammatory Syndrome Over 20 Years (not accounting for costs borne by insurer)	
Typical weight loss program [1]	$9/week; $9,360 for 20 years
Cost of general healthcare for diabetic patient [2]	$13,000/year; $260,000 for 20 years
Gastric bypass [3]	$20,000
Hospital admission and treatment for heart failure [3]	$6,258
Cardiac bypass surgery	$50,000
Pacemaker, including implantation, hardware, hospital fees, professional fees, and outpatient care [3]	$22,000
Total approximate cost of Sedentary-Inflammatory Syndrome	$367,618

[1] ConsumerSearch.com
[2] Centers for Disease Control
[3] Health Care Blue Book

Sedentary-Inflammatory Syndrome is a dysfunction caused by lifestyle choices. With awareness can come wiser choices, improved long-term wellness, and vast financial benefit.

Chapter Five
Stress Imbalance Syndrome
(Chronic Stress + Insomnia + Clinical Depression)

The worst thing in the world is to try to sleep and not to.
— *F. Scott Fitzgerald*

We tend to not regard stress or insomnia as medical conditions, but rather as unavoidable aspects of our modern lifestyle. Stress is "just part of life," while insomnia is seen as the simple inability to get some sleep once in a while. Even depression, a serious disease that is the leading cause of disability in the U.S., is too often overlooked. It's hard to take a syndrome seriously, if you don't acknowledge that there is a progression of dysfunction underlying it, or that if it is left untreated, it can progress to a much more serious condition.

These conditions are legitimate causes of BioDebt. Unrelieved emotional and psychological stress may inflict greater damage on the body than any other condition. This is in part because it produces chronic levels of powerful hormones that harm the cardiovascular, nervous, and immune systems, but also because it is not regarded as an illness. Popular ignorance about the dangers of stress turns it into a stealth killer that can trigger Stress Imbalance Syndrome.

Stress Imbalance Syndrome
- Chronic Stress
- Insomnia (Sleep Hormone Dysfunction)
- Depression (Neurochemical Dysfunction)

Based on a solid and growing body of scientific research, we know that the physiological effects of unrelenting stress lead to imbalances and deficiencies in the hormones and neurochemicals that regulate our sleep cycles. This leads to the name of the condition, Stress Imbalance Syndrome. When we are deprived of restorative sleep, it becomes easier to slip into clinical depression or into a self-reinforcing cycle of insomnia and depression that can sap **BioWealth** and destroy quality of life.

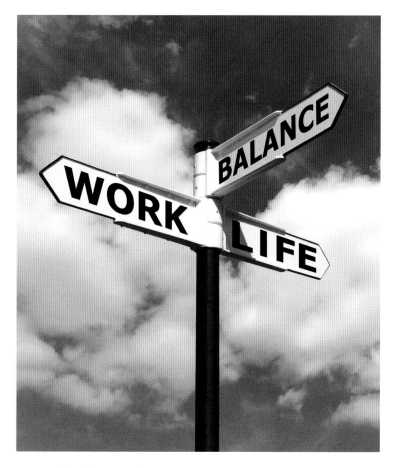

As with Sedentary-Inflammatory Syndrome, there is a clear progression with Stress Imbalance Syndrome from stage to stage, each stage exacerbating the nutritional depletion brought about by the prior stage. Fortunately, this connectivity also points the way to alleviating this nightmarish process and restoring function with nutrition and lifestyle changes. But first, let's explore the stages more closely, starting with stress.

What Dysfunctions?

B Vitamins

B vitamins are destroyed by alcohol, refined sugars, nicotine, and caffeine, so it is not uncommon for people fully engaged in the modern Western lifestyle to be deficient in one or more. Vitamin B6 is a constituent of many amino acids, so low levels can contribute to a deficiency of amino acids that promote sleep. Vitamin B12 deficiency can result in reduced levels of key neurotransmitters, resulting in loss of memory, restlessness, and fatigue. The brain uses Vitamin B1 (thiamine) to convert glucose into fuel, so deficiency can lead to fatigue, depression, irritability, anxiety, and thoughts of suicide. Vitamin B5 (pantothenic acid) is essential for the uptake of amino acids and the neurotransmitter acetylcholine—deficiency can be a factor in certain types of depression. Folic acid is needed for the manufacture of S-adenosyl methionine, or SAM, a coenzyme that preliminary studies suggest may play a role in preventing depression and Alzheimer's disease.

Antioxidants

As cortisol produced by the "stress response" produces free radicals that can damage cellular structures, antioxidant deficiency leads to oxidative damage to cholesterol, cells, and DNA throughout the body.

Amino Acids (Tryptophan)

Tryptophan has been shown to increase levels of the calming neurotransmitter serotonin and the sleep-inducing hormone melatonin. Logically, a deficiency of this amino acid can produce deficiencies in both molecules, leading to sleep disruption.

Omega-3 Fatty Acids

In addition to their anti-inflammatory properties, Omega-3 fatty acids are also important for memory, cognitive performance, and overall brain function, due to their role as the building blocks of brain cell membranes and of myelin, the protective sheath that covers neurons. Symptoms of Omega-3 fatty acids deficiency include extreme fatigue, mood swings, and depression.

Chromium

The chronic intake of sugar and refined starches leads to chromium depletion and chronically elevated levels of insulin. Chromium deficiency impairs cellular insulin sensitivity and blood sugar metabolism, which can affect energy levels and contribute to fatigue and depression.

Supportive Nutrients

Green Tea contains powerful antioxidants called polyphenols which have been shown to protect sensitive brain structures and boost the availability of the signaling agent dopamine.

Amino Acids (Theanine) is an amino acid which helps create mental calmness.

Stage 1: Stress

Research has linked chronic stress to depression. Scientists first noticed the link between cortisol (the main stress hormone) and depression in patients with Cushing's Syndrome, a disease caused by an excess production of cortisol. They found that an excess of cortisol could cause symptoms commonly seen in severe depression. Even more revealing, in a number of published studies patients with Cushing's Syndrome who received treatment that lowered cortisol levels experienced decreased depression symptoms including feelings of fatigue, feelings of worthlessness, impaired concentration, insomnia or excessive sleeping, diminished interest in activities, thoughts of death or suicide, or weight loss or gain. In the largest study, of 176 patients, 73% of the depressed patients showed improvements in their depressive symptoms with reduced cortisol levels. The link between stress and depression seems clear.

Stress is the body's normal, healthy response to a threat. In a survival situation, the brain tells the endocrine system to dump massive quantities of two powerful hormones—epinephrine and cortisol—into the body. These chemicals channel energy to the muscles, increase blood pressure and body temperature, speed up thinking, and help us escape the threat. That's what an "adrenaline rush" is.

Here's the key: the body's stress response mechanism evolved to activate, help us survive danger, and then shut down. It was never meant to be switched on 24 hours a day, 7 days a week. But with recession, job losses, war, crime, traffic, and the upheaval of modern life, that system is regularly flooding our bodies with cortisol and epinephrine. At high levels, these stress chemicals wreak havoc on the body, including:

- Increased fat deposits around the middle, leading to higher cholesterol levels, insulin resistance, and diabetes.
- Elevated blood pressure, causing damage to blood vessels and the heart muscle, raising the risk of cardiovascular dysfunction.
- Irritable bowel syndrome.
- Immune system damage, leaving the body vulnerable to infections and cancer.

In struggling to prevent and repair this ongoing damage, the body's systems deplete vital nutrients such as B Vitamins and the antioxidant Vitamin C. The compensatory depletion that begins with stress plays out as indicated below, with the hyper-stressed individual often exhibiting deficiencies.

Compensatory Depletion: Stress		
Primary Deficiency	**Secondary Depletion**	**Supportive Nutrients**
B Vitamins Antioxidants	Amino Acids (Tryptophan) Omega-3 Fatty Acids Chromium Picolinate	Green Tea Amino Acids (Theanine)

According to the American Psychological Association (APA), stress is linked to six of the leading causes of death among Americans: cardiovascular disease, cancer, respiratory disease, accidents, cirrhosis of the liver, and suicide.

Stage 2: Insomnia (Sleep Dysfunction)

Part of this epidemic, if it comes, will involve insomnia. The same cultural ethos that makes us regard chronic stress as normal also compels us to look at sleep as an optional event—even as a sign of weakness. The need for sleep is not well understood, but we know that it is essential to virtually every aspect of physical and mental **BioWealth**. Research funded by the U.K.'s Wellcome Trust has identified a link between sleeplessness and paranoid thinking. The study revealed that people in the general population suffering from chronic insomnia were 500% more likely to experience high levels of paranoid thinking than people who were getting enough sleep. More than half the individuals requiring psychiatric services for severe paranoia were also found to have clinical insomnia.

Sleeplessness can be a chronic, biological condition. The process of falling asleep involves a gradual drawing-down of metabolic action.

- Our muscles relax.
- We consume less oxygen.
- Our body temperature drops.
- Brain activity changes as alpha and beta waves, the brainwaves associated with conscious thought, transition into the delta waves indicative of deep sleep.

But if we're stressed out, the release of cortisol blocks these changes, putting us in a state of arousal. This is why it is so difficult to fall asleep if you're worried about money or angry with your boss. The real trouble begins when years of unrelenting stress stimulate chronically-elevated cortisol levels, leaving us hyper-aroused. When that happens, sleep suffers—and even when we do sleep, it's shallow and non-restful.

Hormones Out of Balance

Cortisol is the first hormone involved in this progression. The second is melatonin, which your body needs to regulate your circadian rhythm, which is the mechanism that controls sleep and wakefulness. Melatonin is synthesized from serotonin, one of the "master" neurotransmitters. High levels of cortisol interfere with the serotonin receptors in the brain, throwing off the body's serotonin balance. Our hypothesis, based on extensive review, is that excessive cortisol both inhibits the synthesis of serotonin and *destroys key serotonin-containing neurons in the brain.* That's right: too much stress can actually destroy parts of your brain. This damage results in an imbalance of melatonin, and sleeplessness results.

Once this hormone-depleted state is reached, a vicious downward spiral can result. It's thought by some researchers that sleep loss may begin as an attempt to correct this hormonal imbalance and to cool off the hyper-arousal of body and brain caused by the stress response. However, this unconscious reaction actually starts a cycle of dysfunction. Once a bout of insomnia happens, most people feel frustrated and anxious about getting enough sleep and change their behavior to compensate for sleep loss, by:

- Napping during the day or early evening
- Going to bed early the next night
- Staying in bed later the next morning
- Drinking alcohol as a way to "get to sleep"

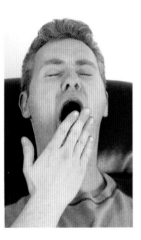

But those behaviors alter the normal sleep mechanism and wind up *perpetuating* insomnia! Things rapidly go downhill from here, as disordered sleep sets off a cascade of symptoms: fatigue, irritability, memory and concentration problems, loss of sex drive, weight loss, loss of interest in social and other activities, and the inability to draw pleasure from them, and so on. Fatigue makes functioning difficult and often wraps the patient in a cloud of pessimism. Conditions are perfect for depression.

Sleeping Keeps Us Young

Even without depression, chronic insomnia can cause serious BioDebt. Experts estimate that the average person needs 8.4 hours of sleep per night. Yet the National Sleep Foundation says that more than half of those who responded to a survey said they experienced symptoms of insomnia, while 35% said they experienced such symptoms every night or most nights. Not getting enough sleep throws many of our key hormones—serotonin, leptin, prolactin, and thyroid—out of whack. In fact, according to a study conducted by the University of Chicago and colleagues in Belgium, insomnia-induced hormone changes are very similar to the processes associated with aging, including a lower production of human growth hormone. In short, insomnia may age us prematurely. Some of the consequences of long-term clinical insomnia are:

- Increased risk of cardiovascular dysfunction and stroke.
- High blood pressure.
- Weight gain.
- Impaired immune function.
- Mood disorders.
- Impaired concentration and memory.
- Decreased enjoyment of relationships.

Insomnia also accelerates the nutritional depletion begun by chronic stress.

Compensatory Depletion: Insomnia		
Primary Deficiency	**Secondary Depletion**	**Supportive Nutrients**
B Vitamins	Omega-3 Fatty Acids	Amino Acids (Theanine)
Antioxidants	Chromium	
Amino Acids (Tryptophan)		

And there's more: the National Highway Safety Administration says that more than 1,500 highway fatalities and 71,000 injuries each year can be blamed on sleep-deprived and drowsy motorists. In total, sleeplessness-related health problems cost a staggering $16 billion per year. Few are more serious or frightening than clinical depression.

Stage 3: Depression (Neurochemical Dysfunction)

Insomnia and depression can be a chicken-egg situation, because depression can also be a cause of sleeplessness. But it's clear that a chronic lack of sleep and the resulting hormonal chaos can bring about fluctuations in key neurotransmitters and produce mood disorders, including life-threatening depression. In disrupting the brain and serving as a stressor by itself, sleep loss renders people even more vulnerable to depression and precipitates the onset of depressive episodes.

About 80% of depressed patients experience insomnia, according to mental health professionals. A 1996 study conducted by Breslau, Roth, Rosenthal and Andreski monitored 1,200 young adults for three years and found that those with insomnia were 400% more likely to develop a new major episode of depression. There remains little question that, aside from all the other ways it can damage the heart, brain, immune system, and overall health, insomnia is a profound risk factor for depression.

Depression is a serious dysfunction. According to the National Institutes of Health and the National Institute of Mental Health, it's estimated that 9.8% of Americans over age 18 suffer from some sort of depressive disorder. This is a staggering total of approximately 22 million people, two-thirds of them women.

It is also impossible to ignore the fiscal consequences. The direct and indirect costs of depression are staggering—an estimated $44 billion of costs or more annually for the U.S. economy. It is hardly surprising that the bestselling pharmaceutical prescriptions in the country are antidepressant drugs like Prozac™ and Paxil™.

Depression shatters lives. Its symptoms can cause difficulty concentrating, fatigue, feelings of worthlessness or helplessness, pessimism, loss of appetite, loss of interest in once-beloved activities, irritability, persistent pain, suicidal thoughts, and suicide attempts. This is aggravated by the fact that the desire to seek and follow through with treatment is often blunted by profound feelings of sadness, hopelessness, and lethargy. Far more than "the blues," true clinical depression is a dangerous condition that is notoriously difficult to treat.

Insomnia's link to depression is complex. Depression changes Rapid Eye Movement (REM), the sleep that is the hallmark of dreaming and restorative rest. Disordered REM sleep is a strong indicator of depression. Depressive people often "rush" into REM sleep; into a dream state that can be traumatic. Early-stage insomnia may actually be the brain's effort to correct depression. Evidence has shown that extended wakefulness actually increases activity of the serotonin system, as well as increasing the release of dopamine, the "reward hormone" which is also linked to depression.

But insomnia isn't a cure for depression. Serotonin—the third card in our hormonal poker hand—is the key. Twenty-five percent of people with depression exhibit low levels of serotonin metabolism. This is how differing serotonin levels make you feel:

Normal Serotonin Levels
- You feel good.
- You sleep and eat well.
- You awake refreshed and energized.

Low Serotonin Levels
- You feel lethargic.
- You can't sleep or sleep too much.
- You lose your appetite.
- You stop taking pleasure in things.
- You feel hopeless.

Notice any similarities with clinical depression? You should. Serotonin is synthesized in the brain, but also in the digestive tract. This is why what you eat and how well you digest your food are crucial to how you feel. Of course, chronic stress also interferes with normal digestion.

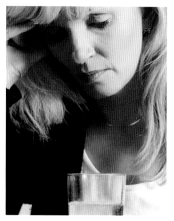

So rather than Stress Imbalance Syndrome being a purely linear progression, it appears that each condition reinforces the others. Stress leads to insomnia. Insomnia brings on greater stress, even as it opens the door to depression. Depression tightens the grip of insomnia, leading to greater stress, and around and around again. In the end, each dysfunction within this syndrome may inflame the severity of the others in a sort of *pas de trois* of disability.

Compensatory Depletion: Depression		
Primary Deficiency	**Secondary Depletion**	**Supportive Nutrients**
B Vitamins Antioxidants Amino Acids (Tryptophan) Omega-3 Fatty Acids Chromium	⬅	Amino Acids (Theanine)

Preventing Stress Imbalance Syndrome

We can all choose our individual stress response and how we manage stress. Stress is unavoidable at times, but we can develop coping skills and devices to manage the effects of stress on our lives and prevent Stress Imbalance Syndrome before it begins. Examples of some coping skills and devices would be the following:

- We consciously redirect our responses to stressful events and develop skills to cope with stress in healthy ways.
- Because the opposite of a hyper-aroused stressful state is a relaxed, calm state, we enjoy more restful, restorative sleep.
- We understand that good sleep is of great help in preventing anxiety, cognitive difficulties, and mood swings that can lead to depression.

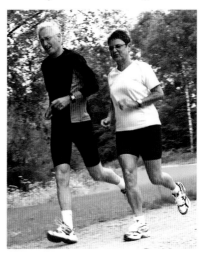

We are not suggesting that reducing stress and insomnia will cure all cases of depression. The literature supports the idea that chemical events in the brain, life events, and genetics can all also play a role in the onset of depression. But, given the deep link to insomnia, an optimized lifestyle with good dietary and supplementation measures could reverse or prevent the cycle that leads to depressive dysfunction from ever beginning. Here are some of the holistic, preventive actions you can take:

Lifestyle Modifications

Make sleep a priority—The human sleep cycle is not naturally 16 hours off, 8 hours on. We nap, doze, wake up, get things done, and then drop off again. Discover your own sleep pattern and stop trying to force your body into a prescribed sleep "form." Add sleep where you can during the day with naps, rest breaks, daydreaming, and anything else that allows your mind to drift and recuperate, even if it does not involve sleep. Finally, make sleep a priority at night. Remove all non-sleep activities from your bedroom. Create a physical, olfactory, visual, and auditory environment that is conducive to rest, relaxation, and deep sleep. Give yourself a regular bedtime, and develop a bedtime ritual that begins at that time, getting your body and mind ready for sleep.

Exercise—Exercise releases beneficial mood-improving hormones and also reduces the impact of stress on the body by dilating blood vessels, damping inflammation, burning excess energy, and even by encouraging the development of new neural connections in the brain.

Meditate—Regular meditation has a profoundly positive effect on the immune system. Mindfulness meditation is relatively easy to learn, though there are dozens of different styles of meditation. Also consider meditative exercise such as yoga or Tai Chi.

Dietary Modifications

Avoid caffeine, alcohol, and sugar—Caffeine keeps you up and prevents restful sleep. Alcohol stimulates the secretion of adrenaline, resulting in nervous tension, irritability, and insomnia. Sugar creates worthless short-term energy and stresses the adrenals, so when you come off the "sugar high," you feel depressed and lethargic.

Eat more fiber—Stress can cause digestive distress, so eating fiber in whole grains, vegetables, and fruits can help keep your digestive habits regular.

Eat more vegetables—This can increase your brain's production of serotonin, a neurotransmitter vital to mood, as well as one leading to better absorption of the important amino acid L-tryptophan. Also, more fruit and vegetable consumption helps support your immune system.

Power Nutrient Supplements

Amino Acids—Stress and resulting insomnia can disrupt the normal levels of key amino acids in the dopamine, norephrine, and serotonin systems, which are vital to maintaining mood and cognitive function. Supplementing with key amino acids such as L-tryptophan (which the body uses to synthesize serotonin) and theanine (which reduces mental and physical stress, may produce feelings of relaxation, and improves cognition and mood) may help prevent the depletion of vital neuro-transmitters.

Omega-3 Fatty Acids—Omega-3 fatty acids have been shown to improve brain function. In particular, DHA is essential for the healthy function of brain cell mem-branes. Some researchers think that disorders like depression, bipolar disorder, and schizophrenia may be due in large part to a deficiency of these Omega-3 fatty acids.

Chromium Picolinate—Researchers at Duke University found that this mineral can reduce depressive symptoms, possibly by increasing insulin sensitivity, and therefore improving the loss of appetite and energy that many depression suffer-ers experience.

Green Tea—According to a study by University College London researchers, drink-ing tea lowers stress hormone levels. In addition, the act of drinking tea is relaxing and can help calm the mind.

Antioxidants—High levels of stress hormones can promote inflammation and damage to sensitive neurological systems. Antioxidants have been shown to pro-vide protection for these structures.

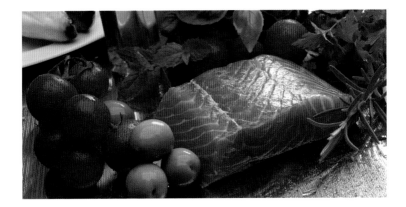

What It Can Cost

We've already discussed the staggering cost of treating clinical depression, from hospitalization and drugs to lost productivity. But there are further costs to Stress Imbalance Syndrome, many of them subtler than the obvious costs of Sedentary-Inflammatory Syndrome. But they remain high and rising and inflict a massive fiscal burden on both individuals and society.

Hypothetical Total Costs of Managing Stress Imbalance Syndrome Over 20 Years (not accounting for costs borne by insurer)	
Hypertension medication [1]	$100/month; $24,000 over 20 years
Hospitalization for severe or chronic headache [1]	$3,600
Mental health counseling [1]	$75/session once per week; $75,000 over 20 years
Sleep aid [2]	$16,560
Depression drugs (Prozac, etc.) [2]	$67,200
Hospitalization for depression [3]	$21,800
Total approximate cost of Stress Imbalance Syndrome	$208,160

[1] *Health Care Blue Book*
[2] Blue Cross/Blue Shield of Tennessee
[3] *Psychiatric Services,* February 2000

Like our first syndrome, Stress Imbalance Syndrome is a matter of lifestyle choice. This offers hope that depression can be reversed and quality of life restored by the replenishment of key nutrients and some wise lifestyle decisions. With any dysfunction, an understanding of its true nature is the key to **BioWealth**.

Chapter Six
Bone Dysfunction Syndrome
(Osteoporosis + Osteoarthritis)

*"I am interested in physical medicine because my father was.
I am interested in medical research because I believe in it.
I am interested in arthritis because I have it."*
— Bernard M. Baruch, American Economist
and adviser to U.S. presidents

Neither of these dysfunctions of the bones and joints is directly life threatening, but they can have a terrible impact on the quality of life. Osteoporosis and osteoarthritis also differ from the other syndromes in a vital way. The others have a typical progression that looks like this:

Obesity ➡ Diabetes ➡ Cardiovascular Dysfunction
Stress ➡ Insomnia ➡ Clinical Depression

Bone Dysfunction Syndrome maps in a different way:

Nutritional Deficiency

Osteoarthritis   Osteoporosis

Where the other syndromes follow a fairly linear progression, this syndrome takes on more of a "tree root" structure. Instead of osteoporosis leading directly to osteoarthritis or the other way around, they share the same common taproot of nutritional deficiency, most significantly a lack of Vitamin D and Omega-3 fatty acids. From this single source spring two diseases that have much in common, are often found in the same patients, and can exacerbate the severity of each other. So nutritional deficiency leads to a progressive, self-reinforcing disease process that impacts bone and joint health and can bring chronic pain, reduced mobility, increased risk of fractures, reduced quality of life and even a lower life expectancy.

What Dysfunctions?

Vitamin D

In addition to supporting the uptake of calcium necessary for bone health and the formation of new bone mass, Vitamin D has been shown to play a role in the synthesis of synovial fluid, the body's joint lubricant. Vitamin D deficiency can result in poor production of new bone, bone density loss, and poor joint lubrication, leading to pain and the development of such symptoms as bone spurs and joint swelling.

Omega-3 Fatty Acids

Because of their powerful anti-inflammatory effects (as well as research showing that they may reduce levels of a cartilage-destroying enzyme), a deficiency in Omega-3 Fatty Acids can make the joints more vulnerable to swelling and stiffness and accelerate cartilage loss.

Glucosamine

Low levels of glucosamine can hamper the body's ability to rebuild damaged cartilage and thus accelerate the effects of osteoarthritis.

Minerals (Calcium, Magnesium)

A deficiency of calcium, the most abundant mineral in the body, is linked to poor levels of bone remineralization and bone repair, leading to loss of bone density. Magnesium acts as a catalyst, binding calcium and fluorine to build bone. Thus a deficiency in this mineral impairs the body's ability to build new bone.

Supportive Nutrients
Green Tea

Evidence indicates that green tea reduces the impact of inflammatory chemicals common to bone and joint dysfunction.

Pomegranate

Rich in antioxidant flavonoids, pomegranate blocks degradation of cartilage by inflammatory chemicals.

Osteoporosis (Bone Mineralization Dysfunction)

Osteoporosis is the long-term loss of bone tissue that robs bones of their density and leaves them brittle and vulnerable to fractures. It affects approximately 10 million Americans, most of whom are women, and tends to appear more in older people. An estimated 34 million more have *osteopenia*, bone density not low enough to qualify as osteoporosis but indicative of progress *toward* osteoporosis. In its most severe forms, it can cause chronic lower back pain, height loss, and physical deformity such as the infamous "Dowager's Hump" sometimes seen in senior women. Osteoporosis also leaves its sufferers highly susceptible to broken legs and hips, which can be disastrous injuries for the elderly.

There is no clear single cause for this dysfunction, though researchers have identified several common causal factors that can indicate a higher risk:

- Petite, slender frame
- Asian or Caucasian descent
- Being post-menopausal
- Dysmenorrhea (absence of menstrual periods)
- Family history
- Low calcium intake
- Sedentary lifestyle
- Smoking
- Excessive alcohol use

The skeletal system is quite dynamic. Bone mass is being shed and replaced constantly. In people with osteoporosis, this process is inhibited until bone tissue lost through normal means is not replaced at a level that allows the bones to retain their usual strength and resistance to fractures. As you can imagine, the bones that take the greatest impact—the bones in the legs, hips and spine—are the most vulnerable.

Osteoporosis has no obvious symptoms, which makes it a silent condition—until the afflicted person suffers a serious fracture. A very simple, non-invasive test called a Bone Density Test can check for osteoporosis, but too many women do not have this test early enough to arrest its progress. That's unfortunate, because it has some grim financial and social consequences.

- 500,000 people are hospitalized annually for osteoporosis-related problems.
- 180,000 people are placed in nursing homes for the same reasons.
- $18 billion in direct health care costs.

The hip fractures common among patients with advanced osteoporosis can be deadly. When you combine the stress of hospitalization, the loss of mobility, the pain and depression and the dangerous side effects of post-hospitalization drugs, it's not surprising that 20% to 24% of the 300,000 people in the U.S. who break their hips each year die within a year of the injury. This is a serious condition with serious consequences.

Some common prescription drugs can worsen osteoporosis or even cause it in otherwise healthy people. The corticosteroid Prednisone, which is very commonly used to treat asthma as well as immune disorders, can cause bone loss if used over the long term. Also, a class of acid reducing drugs known as "proton pump inhibitors" (including Nexium and Prevacid) can increase the risk of hip fractures. Anti-seizure drugs have also been shown to increase the risk. So risk is all around.

Because Bone Dysfunction Syndrome is not linear, the mechanism of compensatory depletion doesn't apply in the same way here. However, people with osteoporosis do tend to be deficient in certain nutrients.

Compensatory Depletion: Osteoporosis	
Primary Deficiency	Supportive Nutrients
Vitamin D	Green Tea
Omega-3 Fatty Acids	
Minerals (Calcium, Magnesium)	Antioxidants

Osteoarthritis (Connective Tissue Dysfunction)

Osteoarthritis is a dysfunction of the joints. There are more than 100 types of arthritis, but the one most identified with old age and joint pain is osteoarthritis. Osteoarthritis is a localized, degenerative condition in which the cartilage that cushions the joints is worn away over time. For years, we have assumed that the main cause of arthritis was strenuous activity that pounded the joints, particularly the knees: running, hiking, working construction, playing sports and so on. However, this turns out not to be the case. Athletic activity is beneficial to the joints as it is for every other part of the body.

Barring a traumatic joint injury, the most likely cause of osteoarthritis is obesity. Carrying extra weight for decades, without the therapeutic effects of regular exercise, appears to gradually wear away cartilage and damage bone, leading to pain. In fact, research has shown that the people in the top 20% of the population for Body Mass Index (BMI) are 150% to 200% more likely to develop osteoarthritis over a 36-year period than people of lower weight. Even more telling, losing just 10 pounds reduced that risk by 50%.

When osteoarthritis develops, joint bones grate together, bone spurs form, and joints swell, making even ordinary movements painful. The knees, neck, lower back, and the small joints of the hands are the joints most often affected. Osteoarthritis makes movement and simple daily activities excruciating for as many as 20 million Americans. It's seen as an inevitable consequence of aging as cartilage increases in water content while losing protein—and indeed the American College of Rheumatology estimates that 70% of people over age 70 show x-ray evidence of some level of arthritis. But is it inevitable?

Like osteoporosis, osteoarthritis is not directly a fatal condition. However, it makes daily tasks and mobility excruciatingly painful for millions, and therein lies its threat. We did not evolve to be sedentary creatures. We are beings of movement, designed to walk and run and swim and bike. We thrive on perspiration, elevated heart rate and working muscles. When joint pain robs us of that mobility, we gain weight, suffer from mood disorders, and become subject to more BioDebt. Osteoarthritis of the knee is the leading cause of chronic disability in the elderly in developed countries, with an estimated $60 billion economic impact in the U.S. It's estimated to negatively impact the quality of life for more than 20 million Americans, most of them over 55.

As with osteoporosis, those with osteoarthritis appear to be deficient in certain nutrients:

Compensatory Depletion: Osteoarthritis	
Primary Deficiency	**Supportive Nutrients**
Vitamin D	Green Tea
Glucosamine	Pomegranate
	Antioxidants

The Link Between Osteoarthritis and Osteoporosis

Osteoporosis does not directly bring about osteoarthritis, nor does the reverse appear to happen. However, it is becoming clear that there are links. Several long-term studies of both osteoarthritis and osteoporosis—including the Chingford Study, a long-term study of 1,000 women in the U.K. funded by the Arthritis Research Campaign—suggest that osteoarthritis may be a dysfunction of the bone as well as the cartilage, meaning that the two conditions have unhealthy bone in common. There is some speculation that both diseases are due in great part to the body's being too acidic—that is, being out of pH balance. As a result, these acids damage many areas of the body, including the bones and cartilage. Ours is a different but well-supported theory of the connection between these two conditions, and in fact this book may be the first time this theory has been articulated by medical professionals in a major published work.

The common link between osteoporosis and osteoarthritis is that both arise primarily from a chronic deficiency of Vitamin D.

As we will discuss in greater detail in the Power Nutrient chapter on Vitamin D, this formerly humble vitamin has become a superstar. You know it as the "healthy teeth and healthy bones" vitamin, because it increases the body's ability to absorb calcium and phosphorus, which are needed for bone mineralization,

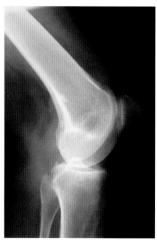

growth and repair. But new studies have shown that Vitamin D is a kind of wonder drug. New research is telling us that Vitamin D can reduce cancer risk, prevent some heart attacks in men, reduce the death rate from all health causes over an eight-year period, and according to 2009 research released by Tufts University, appears to be linked to lower fasting blood sugar levels and better insulin sensitivity. There is even research showing that Vitamin D may protect against immune system disorders, infections like tuberculosis, and perhaps mental illnesses including schizophrenia.

Add osteoarthritis and osteoporosis to the list. This is supported by a growing body of scientific evidence.

- A study from Tufts New England Medical Center that reveals that low Vitamin D levels may cause increased knee pain and difficulty walking in people who already have osteoarthritis.
- According to a Harvard Medical School study, a substantial percentage of women undergoing surgery for osteoarthritis of the hip had both osteoporosis and a deficiency of Vitamin D.
- Research published in 1996 in the *Annals of Internal Medicine*, the result of a study on 556 patients, suggests that low levels of Vitamin D are associated with an increased risk of osteoarthritis, including the formation of bone spurs and cartilage loss.
- Several studies suggest that Vitamin D reduces inflammation. Dr. James Dowd, of the Arthritis Institute of Michigan, has prescribed large doses of Vitamin D to his patients and claims to see amazing results with reduced pain and increased mobility.
- A 2004 study from Boston University showed that not only do Vitamin D deficiencies appear to increase the risk of severe knee osteoarthritis, but also that increasing Vitamin D levels improves muscle strength and physical function for patients with knee osteoarthritis.

It's been known for some time that deficiencies in Vitamin D, calcium, phosphorus and magnesium increase the risk of osteoporosis. But Vitamin D is also a factor in the development of osteoarthritis. Fail to get enough of it and you raise your risk of the disease. Get sufficient doses and you reduce your risk.

Age, smoking, excessive alcohol use, sedentary lifestyle, and genetic history are all risk factors for osteoporosis and osteoarthritis. But Vitamin D appears to be the nutritional common link that bridges the cause-effect gap and shows us a single therapeutic step that may prevent or reduce the severity of both conditions.

Preventing Bone Dysfunction Syndrome

We've mentioned the risks of some osteoporosis drugs, and arthritis drugs also come with their risk factors. Many common pain relievers called non-steroidal anti-inflammatory drugs, or NSAIDs, such as ibuprofen and naproxen, have been linked to increased blood pressure in men, while aspirin can cause stomach problems and bleeding. Prescription analgesics like Vioxx™ and Celebrex™ have been linked to an increased risk of "adverse cardiovascular events"—legal-speak for heart attacks.

Fortunately, you have holistic, systemic options that can prevent these bone dysfunctions and in some cases reduce their severity and even reverse their progression. From a lifestyle perspective, the most important advice is to exercise and control your weight. Exercise stimulates the bones to build new mass, strengthens the muscles around afflicted joints, helps reduce joint inflammation and resulting pain, and replenishes the body's natural supply of lubricant. It also helps prevent weight gain that can increase the strain on joints.

Strength training, especially involving the muscles of the back and spine, can help prevent compression fractures in the spinal column as well as stooped posture. Weight-bearing aerobic exercise such as dancing, walking and stair climbing acts on the bones of the legs and hips to increase bone mass and prevent bone loss. But there is more you can do.

Dietary Modifications

Reduce foods like simple sugars and carbohydrates, which induce joint inflammation and promote weight gain.

Eat more foods rich in calcium, magnesium and Vitamin D—milk, yogurt, cheese, tofu, sardines, salmon, green leafy vegetables

Power Nutrient Supplements

Vitamin D—If you can't spend 15 minutes per day in the sunshine, supplements are an excellent way to get enough of this nutrient that confers so many benefits in so many areas of health. Some advocates saying that 2000 International Units (IU) are enough to get all of the vitamin's benefits, and others claim that up to 10,000 IU are needed for the full protective effects against osteoporosis, osteoarthritis, cancer, and heart disease.

Glucosamine—This is a natural compound found in healthy cartilage and often taken in combination with chondroitin. Solid evidence from clinical trials shows that oral glucosamine supplements strengthen cartilage, especially in osteoarthritis of the knee, where the most testing has been done.

Omega-3 Fatty Acids—Omega-3 fatty acids increase calcium absorption in the gut, reduce the amount of calcium wasted in the urine, increase calcium levels in bone, and improve bone strength.

What It Can Cost

Surprisingly, the costs of managing and treating Bone Dysfunction Syndrome, a non-fatal condition, may be greater than any other syndrome we've discussed because it produces such disability and loss of quality of life. Some examples of the possible costs:

Hypothetical Total Costs of Managing Bone Dysfunction Syndrome Over 20 Years (not accounting for costs borne by insurer)	
Osteoporosis drug [1]	$105/month $25,200 over 20 years
Double knee replacement [2]	$21,600
2 hospitalizations for foot and knee fractures [2]	$28,900
Mobility devices—wheelchairs, scooters [3]	$2,250 (assuming 3 devices over 20 years)
Typical home refitting for mobility and safety [4]	$2,500
Total approximate cost of Bone Dysfunction Syndrome	$81,050

[1] Blue Cross/Blue Shield of Tennessee
[2] *Health Care Blue Book*
[3] http://www.scooter.com
[4] National Association of Homebuilders

It's obvious that measures like getting enough exercise and taking minerals and Omega-3 fatty acids are preferable to the cost, pain and disruption of having joints replaced. Fortunately, as with all the syndromes discussed in *Health Is Wealth*, Bone Dysfunction Syndrome responds well to proper nutrient rebalancing and replenishment. This may offer hope for increased mobility and improved quality of life to many people, not just the elderly and obese.

Now, let's move onto the next section of *Health Is Wealth*, where we will dig deeply into the ten Power Nutrients and explain why they are important and how to use them for your optimal wellness and **BioWealth**.

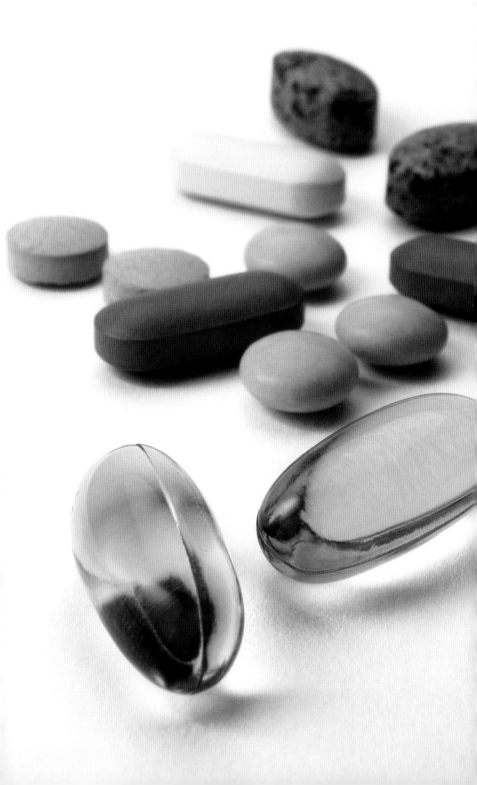

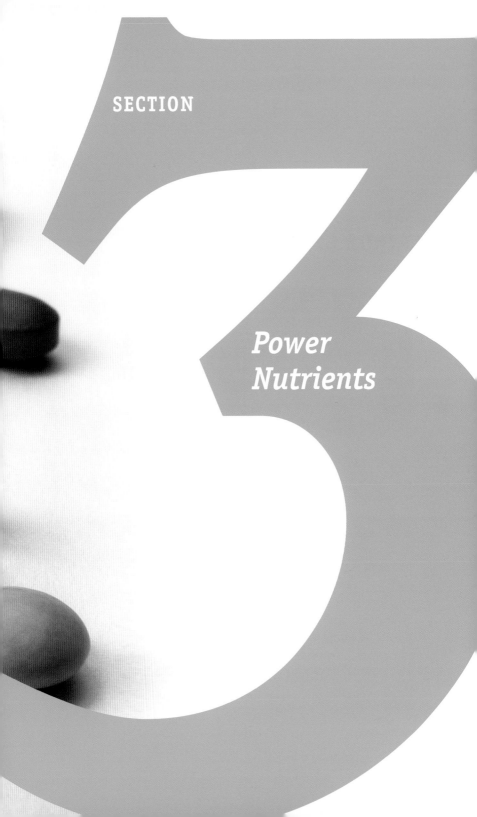

*Power
Nutrients*

Chapter Seven
Alpha Lipoic Acid

Power Facts

✦ Both a water- and fat-soluble antioxidant.
✦ Involved in the conversion of carbohydrates to energy.
✦ Helps improve blood sugar metabolism and insulin sensitivity.
✦ Approved as a drug in Germany for the treatment of diabetic neuropathy.

Few molecules offer more benefits to the body with fewer potential negative side effects than alpha lipoic acid. Alpha lipoic acid is a fatty acid that can be found in every cell; its basic function is to assist the body in converting glucose into usable energy to power the body's normal functions. But as we have discovered, alpha lipoic acid does much more than that.

Alpha lipoic acid is also a potent antioxidant that neutralizes rogue electrons that result from food oxidation, stress and pollution and prevents them from damaging healthy cells. But what makes alpha lipoic acid unique is that it functions in water and fat, unlike common antioxidants Vitamins C and E. Even more impressive, it appears to have power to recycle antioxidants such as Vitamin C and glutathione (often called the master antioxidant) after they have spent their effectiveness by warding off dangerous free radicals. This can make normal dietary intake of other antioxidants far more effective. Finally, alpha lipoic acid is a precursor to glutathione and helps increase the body's levels of this antioxidant.

Scientists first discovered the power of alpha lipoic acid in experiments carried out by the National Institutes of Health in the 1970s. Researchers administered alpha lipoic acid intravenously to 79 people with acute, serious liver damage and 75 of them recovered full liver function. The same research team went on to produce successful results using alpha lipoic acid's ability to alter gene expression to successfully treat pancreatic cancer and lymphoma, extending survival and completely reversing cancer signs and symptoms in one patient's case.

Uses

+ **Potent antioxidant.**
+ **Metabolic enhancer.**
+ **Maintaining blood sugar metabolism and insulin sensitivity.**
+ **Exercise performance aid.**
+ **Supports the treatment of obesity, type 2 diabetes and cardiovascular disease.**

Benefits of Alpha Lipoic Acid

Reducing the Effects of Aging

A major aspect of aging is the cellular damage caused by oxidative stress from free radicals. Antioxidants prevent free radical oxidative damage by "donating" an electron to the free radical and "mopping up" these dangerous molecules. Alpha lipoic acid is one of the most potent and versatile antioxidants. Its capacity to function in both water-soluble and fat-soluble environments means it can access all parts of our cells to neutralize free radicals.

Other research has shown that oxidation damages the mitochondria of the cell, the microscopic system responsible for allowing cells to turn food into energy. Mitochondrial damage is a major factor in aging and degenerative diseases such as cancer, cardiovascular disease, diabetes, immune system failure and cognitive disorders. Alpha lipoic acid, in combination with the amino acid acetyl-L-carnitine, appears to be able to reverse the decay of mitochondria in older people and restore the body's energy conversion functions to levels similar to when they were younger. In other words, alpha lipoic acid may actually reverse some of the core effects of aging.

Benefits of Alpha Lipoic Acid

Diabetes

Insulin produced by the pancreas helps transport glucose and essential amino acids into the body's cells where they can be transformed into usable energy. However, with diabetes or insulin resistance, the body's high levels of blood glucose decrease the efficiency of this transport—and because insulin becomes less effective, greater strain is placed on the pancreas to produce more of it. In pre-diabetics with insulin resistance, this process can often lead to full-blown diabetes.

Research shows that alpha lipoic acid appears to improve glucose uptake in insulin-resistant cells, restoring some of insulin's effectiveness. Several European researchers treated 12 overweight and type 2 diabetic adults averaging 53 years of age with 600 mg of alpha lipoic acid administered orally, twice daily, over four weeks. As a control group, a dozen patients with normal glucose tolerance received the same supplementation. The alpha lipoic acid conclusively increased insulin sensitivity in the diabetic patients over this short time, a very promising result not only for diabetes treatment but also for its prevention.

Another important use of alpha lipoic acid involving type 2 diabetes is in the treatment of peripheral neuropathy—the nerve pain, numbness and tingling often suffered by diabetics. German researchers have found that alpha lipoic acid's antioxidant activity can improve the condition of damaged nerves and ward off further damage. A placebo-controlled study involving 328 diabetic patients showed that a daily intravenous alpha lipoic acid treatment of 600 mg alleviated common symptoms like pain, burning, and itching in the feet for many patients.

Metabolic Syndrome and Heart Disease

Overwhelming evidence now suggests that alpha lipoic acid may not only help the body use glucose with greater efficiency, but may also support proper function of the endothelium—the cellular lining of blood vessels that secretes nitric oxide that improves circulation and cardiovascular health.

A recent analysis of experimental research also shows that alpha lipoic acid can help relieve several components of metabolic syndrome by reducing blood pressure and insulin resistance, improving cholesterol and triglyceride levels, and controlling weight. Additionally, a study of 36 patients with coronary artery disease revealed that a combination of alpha lipoic acid and acetyl-L-carnitine lowers blood pressure and improves endothelial function. Alpha lipoic acid may be a powerful supplemental tool for supporting healthy blood pressure and vascular health.

It appears possible that alpha lipoic acid may also have a protective value in preventing atherosclerosis, or hardening of the arteries. A group of 26 scientists investigated whether alpha lipoic acid therapy inhibits atherosclerosis in mice, and discovered that supplementation significantly reduced atherosclerotic lesion formation in large blood vessels. There is also evidence that alpha lipoic acid has some benefits for controlling body weight. Studies in mice and rats have shown that supplementation reduces the body's ability to accumulate fat and can even reduce diabetes risk by lowering triglyceride levels. This evidence points to tremendous potential benefits for alpha lipoic acid as an agent for preventing what we call Sedentary-Inflammatory Syndrome.

Alzheimer's Disease and Parkinson's Disease

Alpha lipoic acid also appears to have a beneficial effect on cognitive function and brain health. It can cross the blood-brain barrier (a layer of vessels and cells that prevents most substances, including many drugs, from reaching vital brain tissue) and pass into the brain. It is thought to protect brain and nerve tissue by preventing damage by free radicals. This may also protect the brain against the accumulation of beta amyloid plaques, thought to be the major cause of Alzheimer's disease.

In a study of 43 Alzheimer's disease patients extended over four years, researchers found that daily supplementation with 600 mg of alpha lipoic acid along with the neurotransmitter acetylcholinesterase stabilized patients' cognitive functions and drastically reduced the speed of the disease's progression. Other researchers have found that alpha lipoic acid may increase the brain's production of the vital neurotransmitter acetylcholine, which is deficient in people with Alzheimer's disease.

Parkinson's disease may also respond well to alpha lipoic acid supplementation. Early studies show that alpha lipoic acid may prevent the oxidative stress that can damage nerve cells in the substantia nigra, an area of the brain affected by

Parkinson's, causing many of the motor impairments brought on by the disease. By increasing glutathione levels and protecting mitochondria, alpha lipoic acid appears to reduce damage to neural tissues and protect against future damage.

Vision

In several studies, alpha lipoic acid has been found to increase antioxidant enzymes in the eye, protecting against oxidative damage and curbing cataract formation. In a study of patients with "open angle" glaucoma, daily alpha lipoic acid supplementation improved visual function versus control patients who did not receive the supplement. Finally, animal studies indicate that a combination of alpha lipoic acid and Vitamin E appears to prevent the retinal cell death that signals the onset of retinitis pigmentosa.

Nutrient Connections

Research suggests that alpha lipoic acid may exert a "sparing effect" on some antioxidants, including Vitamins C and E. Even after these antioxidants have exhausted their potential to neutralize free radicals at the cellular level, alpha lipoic acid may recharge the molecules to allow them to continue with their protective action. Acetyl-L-carnitine, a modified amino acid, also works cooperatively with alpha lipoic acid.

Interactions

Alpha lipoic acid is extremely safe, but because it can enhance glucose metabolism it should be used appropriately in combination with any diabetes medications.

Recommended Supplementation

- 20 to 50 mg daily for antioxidant protection
- 300 to 600 mg daily for diabetics and cardiovascular dysfunction

Chapter Eight

Amino Acids

Power Facts

✦ The basic building blocks of all proteins.
✦ Some can be made by biological processes; some must be provided through diet or supplementation.
✦ Amino acids that cannot be synthesized are called *essential* and must be obtained from food.
✦ Essential amino acids include lysine, phenylalanine, tryptophan, arginine, tryptophan and histidine.
✦ Non-essential amino acids include alanine, asparagine, aspartate, cysteine, glutamine, glycine, and proline.

You are made of amino acids. These organic compounds are the basic building blocks of life, combining into peptide and polypeptide chains to form the proteins that in turn form your muscles, organs, brain and beyond. It is not surprising that optimal health would depend in great part on refueling the body with a regular and consistent infusion of essential amino acids.

The body uses about 20 standard amino acids in nearly infinite combinations to synthesize the tens of thousands of different proteins that form you. What's more, hundreds of non-protein amino acids are found in nature, and also have vital roles to play, such as the neurotransmitter GABA. Also, many amino acids are used to synthesize other molecules. As we discussed in Chapter 5, tryptophan is the precursor of the neurotransmitter serotonin.

Of the 20 core amino acids used by the body, some can be made by the body, while others must be provided through diet or supplementation. Amino acids that cannot be synthesized are called *essential* and must be obtained from food or from dietary supplements.

Many of us supplement with vitamin and mineral tablets and fewer with herbals or essential nutrients such as Omega-3 fatty acids; however, a relative scarcity of individuals know the effects that insufficiency of certain amino acids can have on their health, or that they should be supplementing with amino acids or that doing so is even possible.

What makes amino acids even more problematic is that for children, the non-essential amino acids cysteine, taurine, tyrosine, histidine and arginine are semi-essential because their bodies have not fully developed the ability to synthesize these molecules. Yet non-essential amino acids can yield important benefits. For example, arginine supplementation is known to increase the body's production of nitric oxide, which dilates blood vessels, lowers blood pressure, prevents cholesterol buildup and protects against heart disease. This is why it is so vital, as we work to address the chronic effects of Nutrient Deficiency Syndrome, that amino acid supplementation becomes a priority for health optimization.

Uses

The wide range of functions performed by various amino acids precludes us from listing all their uses here. Instead, we will present the key benefits of some of the most important amino acids from the perspective of supplementation to prevent Nutrient Deficiency Syndrome.

Benefits of Amino Acids

Following are the positive effects that optimal supplemental levels of what we consider to be the most important amino acids have on the body.

Arginine

Our bodies can produce arginine, but not at sufficient levels to get its most dramatic benefits. Individuals who suffer from poor nutrition or have certain

Benefits of Amino Acids

physical conditions are advised to supplement their diet with arginine or increase the intake of foods containing arginine.

Arginine plays an important role in the healing wounds, removing ammonia from the body, supporting the immune function, and the release of hormones. Arginine is the sole precursor to the synthesis of nitric oxide, which as we have discussed, contributes to improved blood pressure, reduced "bad" cholesterol, and a healthier cardiovascular system. A 2008 study published in the *Journal of Nutrition* revealed that arginine reduced fat gain and increased muscle mass gain in rats, a development that could lead to its use in controlling obesity.

Other benefits and functions attributed to oral ingestion of arginine include:

- Stimulation of the release of the most important anti-aging hormones.
- Improved immune function.
- Reduced healing time for injuries, particularly bones.
- Reduced risk of heart disease.
- Increased muscle mass.
- Reduced body fat.
- Improved insulin sensitivity.
- Decreased blood pressure.
- Alleviation of male infertility by improving sperm production and motility.
- Increased circulation throughout the body, including the sex organs.

Tyrosine

Tyrosine is one of the standard 20 amino acids used by cells to synthesize proteins. The word "tyrosine" is from the Greek "tyros" meaning cheese, as it was first discovered in 1846 by a German chemist in the protein casing of cheese. Aside from being a building block for protein, tyrosine has a special role in *signal transduction*, the process by which a cell converts one kind of stimulus into another.

In humans, tyrosine is synthesized from the amino acid phenylalanine, which is derived from food. In the adrenal gland, tyrosine is then converted to levodopa through an enzyme reaction. Levodopa is involved in the synthesis of vital neurotransmitters like dopamine, epinephrine and nor-epinephrine. The thyroid hormones T3 and T4 are also derived from tyrosine.

Benefits of Amino Acids

A number of studies have found tyrosine to be useful during conditions of stress, fatigue, work, sleep deprivation, and where elevated stress hormone levels are observed. Research has also looked at the role of tyrosine in stress-induced weight loss and in its ability to improve cognitive and physical performance. Tyrosine does not seem to have any significant effect on mood, cognitive ability or physical performance under normal circumstances.

Tryptophan

Tryptophan is one of the twenty standard amino acids, as well as an essential amino acid in the human diet. Tryptophan functions as a biochemical precursor for the following compounds:

- Serotonin, a neurotransmitter, is synthesized from tryptophan hydroxylase. Serotonin in turn can be converted to melatonin.
- Niacin is synthesized from tryptophan.

Some early research indicates that tryptophan may have some role to play in wound healing. A small 2008 study carried out by Balmain Hospital in New South Wales, Australia, revealed that 89% of hospital patients with wounds were deficient in tryptophan (as well as another amino acid, histidine).

Many people find tryptophan to be a safe and reasonably effective sleep aid, probably due to its ability to increase levels of serotonin, a calming neurotransmitter. Serotonin is also integral to the manufacture of melatonin, a sleep-inducing hormone secreted by the pineal gland in response to darkness. Clinical research confirms tryptophan's effectiveness as a sleep aid and for a growing variety of other conditions typically associated with low serotonin levels, including premenstrual dysphoric disorder and seasonal affective disorder, in which a person suffers depressive symptoms in response to the changes that accompany the transition into the dark winter months. In particular, tryptophan has shown promise as a natural antidepressant.

Taurine

Taurine, a conditionally essential amino acid, is a major constituent of the digestive secretion bile and it can be found in lesser amounts in other tissues in the human body.

Benefits of Amino Acids

Studies completed in laboratory animals have demonstrated multiple physiological roles for taurine. Obese mice showed reduced levels of taurine, a factor that may have contributed to their weight gain. Taurine in increased levels has also been shown to decrease weight and blood sugar in studies of diabetic rats. Recent studies have also shown that boosted levels of taurine can influence—and possibly reverse—defects in nerve blood flow and motor nerve conduction, and improve nerve function in diabetics. According to animal studies, taurine may act as a modulator or anti-anxiety agent in the central nervous system. In recent years, taurine has also been combined with other performance enhancing nutrients, partly due to findings that taurine alleviates muscle fatigue in strenuous workouts and raises exercise capacity.

Lysine

Lysine is an essential amino acid and a necessary building block for all protein in the body. Lysine plays a major role in calcium absorption, building muscle protein, recovering from surgery or sports injuries, and in the body's production of hormones, enzymes and antibodies. Lysine is also highly beneficial to those with herpes simplex infections because it can inhibit viral growth.

Not surprisingly, such a crucial molecule brings with it some serious symptoms of deficiency, including damage to muscle and connective tissues, fatigue, poor concentration, hair loss, and anemia.

Cysteine

Although classified as a non-essential amino acid, cysteine may be essential for infants, the elderly, and individuals with certain metabolic diseases or who suffer from malabsorption syndromes. Cysteine can usually be synthesized by the human body under normal conditions, if a sufficient quantity of the amino acid *methionine* is available.

Cysteine is a powerful detoxifying agent and, usually in concert with aspartic acid and citrulline, helps the body recover from the toxins created by alcohol consumption and tobacco use. Its antioxidant properties typically take the form of the tripeptide *glutathione*, which is synthesized from cysteine. Glutathione carries out three critical functions in the body:

- Strengthens the immune system.
- Acts as the body's chief antioxidant.
- Directs the functions of other antioxidants and helps molecules like Vitamins E and C be more effective at preventing oxidative damage to cells.

Citrulline

Citrulline is made from *ornithine*, in one of the central processes of the urea cycle. The name citrulline is derived from "citrullus," the Latin word for watermelon, from which it was first isolated in 1930.

Citrulline has been shown to have performance-enhancing effects and to reduce muscle fatigue. It is a highly specialized amino acid involved in maintaining nitrogen balance in the body and in supporting metabolism. But the major benefit of citrulline appears to be that it can be converted into arginine, the powerful amino acid that produces nitric oxide, which in turn contributes to cardiovascular health by dilating blood vessels.

Carnitine

Carnitine is biosynthesized from the amino acids lysine and methionine, primarily in the liver and kidneys, in a process that depends on Vitamin C. In cells it is required for the transport of fatty acids into the mitochondria, which in turn generate energy.

In the course of human aging, carnitine concentrations in cells diminish, affecting fatty acid metabolism in various tissues. Bones are particularly affected when carnitine levels fall, because they require continuous function of the osteoblast cells for the maintenance of bone mass. In post-menopausal women, administration of carnitine can increase serum *osteocalcin* concentrations, helping to improve bone density.

Carnitine also produces substantial antioxidant action in the body, providing a protective effect for cell membranes, particularly in the heart muscle and the endothelium. Carnitine also improves glucose disposal, storage, oxidation and usage in people with type 2 diabetes.

Theanine

Theanine (gamma-glutamylethylamide, or 5-N-ethyl-glutamine) is a glutamic acid analog or amino acid derivative commonly found in green tea. Theanine may be used to reduce stress and anxiety without the tranquilizing effects found in many other calming agents. Scientific evidence shows that theanine stimulates the brain's production of alpha waves, making you feel relaxed but alert and not drowsy. Theanine also helps the body produce other calming amino acids, such as dopamine, GABA, and tryptophan. As one might expect from a calming supplement, theanine may be able to lower elevated blood pressure. In the management of stress-based disorders, theanine is one of the most effective amino acids.

Nutrient Connections and Interactions

Because we cover so many amino acids that act on numerous systems of the body and interact with an enormous range of other molecules, listing all possible connections and interactions is space-prohibitive. To learn more about amino acid connections to other nutrients or possible drug or supplement interactions, please visit www.healthiswealththebook.com.

Recommended Supplementation

- **Arginine**—5,000 to 8,000 mg daily for optimal cardiovascular benefits
- **Tyrosine**—1,000 mg daily for mental and physical enhancement and for depression
- **Tryptophan**—500 to 4,000 mg daily for insomnia and depression
- **Taurine**—2,000 mg daily for cardiovascular and metabolic support
- **Lysine**—1,000 to 2,000 mg daily for immune enhancement
- **Cysteine**—250 to1,500 mg daily for antioxidant support
- **Citrulline**—500 to 2,000 mg daily for optimal cardiovascular benefits
- **Carnitine**—1000 to 2,000 mg daily for metabolic support
- **Theanine**—100 to 400 mg daily for calming benefits

Chapter Nine
Antioxidants

Power Facts

✦ Antioxidants are molecules that pair their own electrons with "free radicals," the rogue electrons that can damage cellular structures, neutralizing them.

✦ Antioxidants are considered possible preventive agents for aging, cancer, diabetes, cardiovascular dysfunction and Alzheimer's disease.

✦ Antioxidants increase the effectiveness of nitric oxide, which dilates blood vessels, contributes to a healthy endothelium which helps to prevent cardiovascular dysfunction.

✦ Antioxidants are abundant in foods such as blueberries, açai berries, apples, pomegranates, strawberries, cherries, plums, sweet potatoes, carrots, pecans and green tea.

Antioxidants may be the mightiest nutritional supplements available to us due to their ability to prevent cellular damage and disease. Consumer food products from tea and juice to dark chocolate tout their antioxidant content on their labels.

The amino acid arginine is also made more effective by antioxidants. Not only do antioxidants prevent oxidative damage, they help your body realize a greater cardiovascular benefit from nitric oxide, the chemical that lowers blood pressure, helps keep our arteries flexible, and reduces cholesterol.

Major dietary sources of antioxidants are multi-colored fruits and vegetables (especially berries, apples and plums), some nuts like pecans, beans, teas, coffee, high-cacao dark chocolate, and red wine.

Uses

In this chapter we will focus on four major antioxidants: Vitamin E (tocopherols), Vitamin C, zinc and selenium:

+ Vitamin E—Blood cell and hemoglobin formation, reproduction, free radical protection, reducing cholesterol oxidation, immune function.

+ Vitamin C—Collagen production, iron absorption, free radical protection.

+ Zinc—Immune system maintenance, reproduction, blood coagulation mechanism, thyroid function.

+ Selenium—Supports numerous metabolic pathways, free radical protection and immune function.

Benefits of Antioxidants

Antioxidants have been linked to reduced risk of cardiovascular disease, neurological disease, some cancers, macular degeneration (the leading cause of blindness), immune disorders and may even lead to increased life expectancy.

In a study of 72 middle-aged people published in the *American Journal of Clinical Nutrition*, eating just under a cup of mixed berries daily for eight weeks was associated with increased levels of "good" HDL cholesterol and lowered blood pressure, two of the factors that lead to improved cardiovascular health. The berry blend included strawberries, red raspberries, bilberries, black currants, lingonberries and chokeberries. It may be the diverse collection of polyphenols —health-promoting plant compounds that includes anthocyanins and ellagic acid—that provided the benefits. Polyphenols are also thought to increase levels of nitric oxide. Additional research has shown further benefits.

- A study done at the University of Florida, Gainesville showed that antioxidant supplementation may be effective at reducing vascular damage inflicted by obesity and diabetes.

- A study at Oxford University of people aged 70-74 found that those who consumed increased levels of flavonoid-rich chocolate, coffee and tea had better cognitive function than those who did not. Now those are the kinds of "vice" studies that would have people lining up to participate in research!

- Another study completed at the Department of Food Science and Technology at the Agricultural University of Athens revealed that people who consumed high levels of red wine and raw "green" olive oil (staples of the Mediterranean diet, both rich in antioxidants) had improved function of the endothelium.

Resveratrol (trans-resveratrol) is an antioxidant phytoalexin produced naturally by several plants when under attack by pathogens such as bacteria or fungi. Published studies indicate that resveratrol may be one of the most effective plant extracts for maintaining longevity. Resveratrol is found in the skin of red grapes and is a constituent of red wine and may be one of the antioxidant components that contributes to the French Paradox – the observation that the French suffer a relatively low incidence of coronary heart disease, despite having a diet relatively rich in saturated fats.

Important dietary sources of major antioxidants include:
- Carrots and green leafy vegetables: *carotenoids*
- Berries: *anthocyans*
- Apples, citrus fruits, and tea: *flavonoids*
- Vegetable oils, nuts and avocados: *tocopherols*
- Red wine and red grapes: *resveratrol*, an especially potent antioxidant
- Dark chocolate: *epicatechin*
- Green tea, cinnamon and turmeric: *catechins*
- Radishes and mustard: *isothiocyanates*
- Citrus and strawberries: *Vitamin C*
- Broccoli and Brussels sprouts: *indoles*

Nutrient Connections

The wide and increasing number of antioxidants and the many foods in which they appear make it impossible to reflect all possible combinations of nutrient interactions here. For more information, please visit www.healthiswealththebook.com.

Interactions

Note: the majority of prescription and over-the-counter drug interactions with these antioxidants result in reduced levels of the antioxidant in the body, a reaction that is not inherently dangerous. However, check with your healthcare provider before you supplement with antioxidants if you use any of the following medications:
- Vitamin E levels can be reduced by some cholesterol-lowering medications.
- Vitamin C can interact with aspirin and non-steroidal anti-inflammatory drugs, reducing Vitamin C levels in the body.

Recommended Supplementation

- **Vitamin E** (d-alpha tocopherol/mixed tocopherols)—800 to 1,000 IU daily
- **Vitamin C**—1,000 to 2,000 mg daily
- **Zinc**—15 to 30 mg daily
- **Selenium**—200 mcg daily

Chapter Ten

Chromium Picolinate

Power Facts

✦ In 1959, chromium was first identified as an element that enables the hormone insulin to function properly.

✦ Refined sugars, white flour and a lack of exercise can deplete the body's levels of chromium.

✦ Chromium aids in weight management by promoting the maintenance of lean muscle and the loss of body fat.

✦ Recent research indicates that chromium picolinate can help to decrease cravings for carbohydrate-rich foods.

Chromium is involved in the body's metabolism and storage of fats, proteins and carbohydrates—the three broad categories of nutrients that comprise the diet. Chromium picolinate was first identified in 1959 as a form of chromium that was highly bio-available and that seemed to help enhance the function of insulin. In diabetics or those with insulin resistance, insulin is less effective at transporting sugars, which eventually impairs pancreatic function.

Over the years, there have been many claims made for chromium, which remains an essential yet overlooked mineral. Research has found benefits related to weight loss and overall health. Chromium, in the form of chromium picolinate, bears some additional looking into.

Benefits of Chromium Picolinate

Chromium picolinate can boast an impressive résumé of health benefits, many related to fitness, muscle development and weight loss: lower body weight, reduced risk of obesity and a resulting lower chance of heart disease. Many of these benefits appear related to a higher dietary intake of chromium, not necessarily chromium picolinate. However, picolinate appears to be the easiest form of the mineral for the body to absorb and use.

Reduced Hunger and Calorie Intake

The results of a randomized, double-blind, placebo-controlled clinical study published online in the journal *Diabetes Technology & Therapeutics* have finally confirmed chromium picolinate's importance as a weight control supplement. This placebo-controlled study, carried out by Pennington Biomedical Research Center, the largest academically based nutrition research center in the world, showed that for a group of 48 overweight women who did not have diabetes, an eight-week chromium picolinate supplementation program reduced hunger levels by 24% and reduced the women's food intake by 25% versus the control group. The women also experienced reduced cravings for high-fat foods, suggesting that regular supplementation with the mineral may affect the release of hormones that regulate appetite and satiety, the feeling of being full.

Diabetes Treatment

Chromium is known to enhance the action of insulin in metabolizing blood sugar, and people with type 2 diabetes have been found to be chromium deficient. The overall evidence of a direct benefit of chromium supplementation for diabetics, however, was scant until results from a large 1997 Chinese study were published. In the study, 180 diabetics took either a chromium supplement or a placebo. After 120 days, the blood sugar levels of the people who received 1000 micrograms per day of chromium picolinate were 15% to 19% lower than in the placebo patients. Other markers of long-term glucose control were also improved.

A meta-analysis of recent diabetes-related studies of chromium picolinate revealed that in 13 of the 15 studies, supplementation improved at least one measure of glycemic control. As more studies are completed, it is clear that chromium will become more widely recognized as a vital component of an over-all supplementation strategy for the prevention and treatment of diabetes.

Weight Control

Since 1971, at least 28 clinical studies have looked at chromium supplemen-tation and its effects on cholesterol and triglycerides. Double-blind, placebo-con-trolled studies have shown that chromium picolinate supplementation can help people increase lean body mass, reduce body fat percentage, and reduce overall body weight when part of a healthy fitness and dietary program. One study of obese subjects showed that chromium picolinate supplementation improved overall body composition (more muscle and less fat) even when the subjects were not dieting. In another study of obese patients on very low calorie nutritional programs, the supplementation helped the patients build more lean body mass.

Alleviating Depression Symptoms

Recent research has revealed a surprising potential link between chromium picolinate and the metabolic and biochemical processes behind mood disorders and depressive illness. Dr. Jonathan Davidson of Duke University published findings of his study in which 15 patients with atypical depression were given chromium supplements and exhibited significant improvements in such signal behaviors like hopelessness, hostility, overeating, and fatigue. Most exciting, the chromium picolinate supplementation alleviated all symptoms in 60% of the study's subjects.

Ongoing clinical research is laying the groundwork for a new understanding of chromium picolinate's role in the production, maintenance or effective-ness of neurotransmitters. These vital chemicals, which are depleted as part of the stress-insomnia matrix we discussed earlier, may be linked to chromium in ways not yet clearly understood.

Nutrient Connections

Chromium picolinate can affect or be affected by the following nutrients:

- Vitamin C—Insulin facilitates the transport of Vitamin C into the cell, so reduced insulin resistance may also confer the added benefit of higher Vitamin C antioxidant activity.
- Biotin—Studies suggest that adding biotin to chromium can improve the management of blood sugar levels in type 2 diabetics.
- Vitamin E—Tocopherols like Vitamin E can improve insulin function, enhancing the effects of chromium.
- Manganese—Manganese is an activator or co-factor of many enzymes involved in carbohydrate metabolism, and its presence may further enhance the ability of chromium to regulate blood sugar.

Interactions

None

Recommended Supplementation

- 200 mcg per day as a maintenance dose
- 500 to 1,000 mcg per day for weight management, metabolic syndrome, type 2 diabetes, and cardiovascular dysfunction

Chapter Eleven
Coenzyme Q10

Power Facts

✦ The second most important nutrient in the cardiovascular system after nitric oxide.

✦ Biopsy results show 75% of cardiovascular patients are deficient in CoQ10.

✦ Statin drugs deplete the body of CoQ10.

✦ CoQ10 is found in every plant and animal cell and is concentrated in the human heart.

Coenzyme Q10 (CoQ10) is a vitamin-like substance and an essential component of mitochondria, the energy-producing units of the cells in our bodies. It is involved in the manufacture of ATP, the energy currency for all of our body processes. CoQ10 is like the spark plug in a car engine. Just as the car cannot function without the initial spark, the human body cannot function without CoQ10. First discovered by researchers at the University of Wisconsin in 1957, research has since demonstrated significant benefits from Co Q10 as an antioxidant, and in the treatment of a number of health concerns.

Because CoQ10 facilitates the conversion of fats and sugars into energy, having sufficient levels is essential to virtually all tissues in the body. When there is a deficiency of CoQ10, metabolic function suffers, and tissues with high energetic demands such as the heart, brain and kidneys can suffer damage. An increasing body of scientific evidence is pointing unquestionably toward CoQ10's role as a major player in the nutritional maintenance of optimal health along with other such versatile Power Nutrients as arginine and Omega-3 fatty acids.

Uses

✦ **Energy production—CoQ10 is involved in mitochondrial function and the production of energy from fat.**

✦ **CoQ10 functions as an antioxidant, especially in the cardiovascular system.**

✦ **CoQ10 confers benefits related to obesity, metabolic syndrome, diabetes, cardiovascular dysfunction, immune health, gum disease, and Parkinson's Disease.**

✦ **It affects exercise and sports performance in ways that are only beginning to be understood.**

Benefits of Coenzyme Q10

As with many Power Nutrients, science is discovering that CoQ10 is beneficial to an ever-widening set of health conditions and biological systems. However, the primary therapeutic applications for CoQ10 are cardiovascular diseases such as congestive heart failure and high blood pressure. It is also effective in the management of some cancers, diabetes, periodontal disease, immune deficiency, and as a performance-enhancing agent in athletes. Furthermore, a 2008 study at Purdue University suggests that CoQ10 supplementation may have anti-aging effects.

Cardiovascular Dysfunction

An important yet frequently overlooked component in the overall management of cardiovascular dysfunction is the promotion of a better functioning heart. Degeneration of the heart is seen in most cardiovascular disease. It is the result of repeated insult to the heart by factors such as low oxygen supply, inflammation and free radical damage. CoQ10 can reverse or prevent the degeneration associated with heart damage, and appears to actually enhance the mechanical function of a failing heart. It does so by providing optimal nutrition at the cellular level, and by acting as an antioxidant to ward off further oxidative damage to healthy heart cells.

CoQ10 deficiency is common in cardiac patients. Biopsy results from heart tissue in patients with cardiovascular disease show CoQ10 deficiency in 50 to 75% of these individuals. Correcting CoQ10 deficiency as part of standard treatment by the nation's cardiologists would produce dramatic improvements in cardiovascular function. This idea may be gaining ground; 2009 research from the Healthcare Professionals Impact Study found that 72% of U.S. cardiologists recommended dietary supplements to their patients, including CoQ10 and Omega-3 fatty acids.

Statin drugs are known to deplete CoQ10 levels in the body. What is not well known by many physicians is that normal aging may also result in CoQ10 reduction by as much as 72%. Combined with a 40% reduction in CoQ10 by statin drugs, this dual effect deficiency may cause severe depletion of CoQ10 at the cellular level.

Congestive Heart Failure

Congestive heart failure is always characterized by an energy depletion status as indicated by low ATP and CoQ10 levels in the heart muscle. The main clinical concerns in congestive heart failure are frequent hospitalization, and the high incidence of arrhythmia, fluid in the lungs, and other serious complications. Several studies show that CoQ10 supplementation is extremely effective in the treatment of congestive heart failure.

In a study done by Canterbury Health Laboratories with 236 patients suffering from chronic heart failure, a plasma deficiency of CoQ10 was found to be a reliable predictor of mortality due to heart failure. In other words, low levels of the nutrient are a harbinger of likely death for those with weak cardiac function.

Benefits of Coenzyme Q10

High Blood Pressure

CoQ10 deficiencies are present in approximately 39% percent of patients with high blood pressure. This finding alone suggests the need for CoQ10 supplementation. However, CoQ10 appears to provide benefits beyond correction of a deficiency. In several studies, CoQ10 actually lowered blood pressure. Two studies conducted by a team of Italian researchers in 1992 and 1994 revealed that supplementation with CoQ10 can reduce systolic and diastolic blood pressure by as much as 10%. In addition, 2008 research with 235 pregnant women at the Central University of Ecuador showed that CoQ10 supplementation reduced the incidence of pre-eclampsia (high blood pressure during pregnancy) by nearly 50% versus women given a placebo.

Because people with hypertension who can benefit from CoQ10 are usually deficient in the first place, the effect of CoQ10 on blood pressure is usually not seen for several weeks as levels build back up to normal. Therefore CoQ10 is not a standard anti-hypertensive medication; rather, it augments typical pharmaceuticals such as beta blockers and diuretics.

Diabetes

A study performed at the University of Coimbra in Coimbra, Portugal, showed that for diabetics, supplementation with CoQ10 and alpha-tocopherol (a form of Vitamin E) may reduce complications and damage to the pancreas. It may be that CoQ10 increases the synthesis of CoQ10-dependent enzymes, which in turn enhance carbohydrate metabolism.

Performance Enhancement

Because CoQ10 is involved in energy production, supplementation may enhance physical performance. Studies of CoQ10 supplementation in sedentary individuals as well as athletes have shown improvement in physical function. CoQ10 has been shown to improve heart rate, workload capacity, and oxygen requirements. These improvements were significant and evident after just a few weeks of CoQ10 supplementation. In addition, other research has revealed that CoQ10 may be a factor in obesity and that raising levels may help improve people's ability to lose weight. In a 1984 Dutch study published in *Biomedical and Clinical Aspects of Coenzyme Q10*, 52% of obese test subjects were CoQ10 deficient.

Additionally, research suggests that CoQ10 may prevent periodontal disease and may have anti-cancer properties related to breast cancer. It may also help prevent retinal decline with age, which is a possible cause of age-related macular degeneration, according to research conducted jointly by Columbia University in New York and Peking University in Beijing, China.

Nutrient Connections

- Nitric oxide-forming amino acids arginine and citrulline
- Carnitine
- Essential fatty acids
- Alpha lipoic acid
- Vitamin E

Interactions

Statin drugs deplete the body of CoQ10.

Recommended Supplementation

- Antioxidant support for optimal health – 100 to 200 mg per day
- Obesity, diabetes, cardiovascular dysfunction – 400 mg per day
- Parkinson's disease – 1,200 mg per day

Chapter Twelve
Omega-3 Fatty Acids—
EPA and DHA

Power Facts

✦ A Harvard study found that over 84,000 people die each year from a deficiency of Omega-3 fatty acids.

✦ Experts estimate that nearly 80 percent of the population does not ingest enough Omega-3 fatty acids.

✦ Our cells are surrounded by fatty envelopes, and Omega-3 fatty acids help keep our cell membranes healthy, flexible and functional.

✦ The body uses Omega-3 fatty acids to produce natural anti-inflammatory substances called prostaglandins.

Omega-3 fatty acids are vital lipids that have been on the decline in the average American diet for many years, but are crucial to cardiovascular and brain health. Our bodies cannot make the three most important types of essential fatty acids, EPA (eicosapentaenoic acid), DHA (docosahexaenoic acid) and ALA (alpha-linolenic acid)—so we must get them from our diets, but our ability to do so no longer measures up. This is due in part to our modern food production methods as well as our dietary choices.

Important note: alpha-linolenic acid is found in vegetable sources like flaxseed oil, but it does not have the same potent health benefits as EPA and DHA, which are found in marine sources, hence the common name, "fish oil." In this chapter, we will focus on EPA and DHA. However, since the body converts a small amount of alpha-linolenic acid into EPA, it remains important to maintain sufficient levels of alpha-linolenic acid as well. A healthy intake of fresh vegetables, whole grains and nuts will help to accomplish a healthy intake of alpha-linolenic acid.

Two types of "omega" fatty acids tend to dominate our foods: Omega-3 and Omega-6. Ideally, we need to maintain a balance of these fats, which are both important to wellness. Today, researchers recommend having a dietary Omega-6 to Omega-3 ratio of anywhere from 1:1 to 4:1, meaning that we should consume about one to four times as much Omega-6 fatty acid, found in foods like corn oil and sunflower oil, as Omega-3 fatty acid. However, the typical American has a ratio more on the order of 14:1 to 20:1. This can lead to health problems from increased blood clotting (a risk factor for heart attack and stroke) to immune system suppression. This imbalance is thought to be a crucial factor in our epidemic of heart disease and stroke.

Research from the Center for Genetics, Nutrition and Health indicates that:
> Human beings evolved on a diet with a ratio of Omega-6 to Omega-3 essential fatty acids (EFA) of approximately 1:1 whereas in Western diets the ratio is 15:1-16.7:1. Western diets are deficient in Omega-3 fatty acids, and have excessive amounts of Omega-6 fatty acids compared with the diet on which human beings evolved and their genetic patterns were established. Excessive amounts of Omega-6 polyunsaturated fatty acids (PUFA) and a very high Omega-6:Omega-3 ratio, as is found in today's Western diets, promote the pathogenesis of many diseases, including cardiovascular disease, cancer, and inflammatory and autoimmune diseases, whereas increased levels of Omega-3 (a low Omega-6:Omega-3 ratio) exert suppressive effects. In the secondary prevention of cardiovascular disease, a ratio of 4:1 was associated with a 70% decrease in total mortality. A ratio of 2.5:1 reduced rectal cell proliferation in patients with colorectal cancer, whereas a ratio of 4:1 with the same amount of Omega-3 had no effect. The lower Omega-6:Omega-3 ratio in women with breast cancer was associated with decreased risk. A ratio of 2-3:1 suppressed inflammation in patients with rheumatoid arthritis, and a ratio of 5:1 had a beneficial effect on patients with asthma, whereas a ratio of 10:1 had adverse consequences. These studies indicate that the optimal ratio may vary with the disease under consideration. Therefore, it is quite possible that the therapeutic

dose of Omega-3 fatty acids will depend on the degree of severity of disease resulting from the genetic predisposition. A lower ratio of Omega-6:Omega-3 fatty acids is more desirable in reducing the risk of many of the chronic diseases of high prevalence in Western societies, as well as in the developing countries, that are being exported to the rest of the world.

The goal of dietary change and supplementation is to reset the balance of Omega-3 versus Omega-6 fatty acids by consuming more EPA (eicosapentaenoic acid) and DHA (docosahexaenoic acid). Both are readily found in fish such as tuna, salmon, mackerel, lake trout, herring, sardines, nut oils and algae. Both are powerful anti-inflammatory agents, which forms the core of their health benefits. Researchers are finding increasing evidence for the body's inflammatory response as a root cause of heart disease, cancer and Alzheimer's disease. By countering the inflammatory effects of the modern diet and lifestyle, essential Omega-3 fatty acids appear to lend powerful protection against developing serious health problems.

Because they are present in brain tissues in high concentrations, essential fatty acids are also strongly linked to cognitive and behavioral health. Research shows that infants who do not get enough of them from their mothers in utero are at risk for vision and neural disabilities. For adults, deficiency of essential fatty acids appears in such symptoms as dry skin, irregular heartbeat, mood swings, depression, chronic fatigue and memory problems. DHA is also a major fatty acid in sperm, and comprises 40% of the fatty acids in the brain, and 60% of fatty acids in the retina. This makes it vital for brain and vision health.

Uses

+ **Anti-inflammatory.**
+ **Cell membrane structure and function.**
+ **Hormone production.**
+ **Antioxidant.**
+ **Treatment of obesity, diabetes, cardiovascular dysfunction, and arthritis.**

Benefits of Omega-3 Fatty Acids— EPA and DHA

Cardiovascular Disease

The power of essential fatty acids to stave off cardiovascular disease stems in great part from substituting monounsaturated and polyunsaturated fats (which include Omega-3s) for the dangerous saturated fats and trans fats found in large quantities in the modern diet. Based on a great deal of clinical evidence, consuming EPA and DHA via diet and/or supplementation can reduce blood pressure, lower triglyceride levels, reduce inflammation in the blood vessels (lowering the risk of atherosclerosis) and inhibit the development of arterial plaques that can rupture and lead to blockages and heart attacks.

These findings may indicate why the Mediterranean Diet (rich in fish and healthy oils such as olive oil) offers such cardiovascular benefits. Long-term consumption of high concentrations of EPA and DHA from fish sources and alpha-linolenic acid from sources like walnuts and flax have been shown to reduce bad cholesterol levels even in people who were consuming an otherwise high-fat diet.

Population-based studies also reveal that eating two servings of fish per week reduces the risk of stroke by as much as 50%. In general, essential fatty acids appear to have a powerful beneficial effect on the circulatory system.

Research suggests that Omega-3 EPA and DHA may help reduce the thickness (viscosity) of your blood, relax your blood vessels, and slightly lower your blood pressure. These actions of Omega-3 all help reduce the risk of heart attack and stroke in the following ways:

- When your blood is thinner, blood platelets are less likely to clump together and form clots.
- When your blood vessels are relaxed they allow more blood to flow through.
- When your blood pressure is lowered your heart doesn't have to work as hard.

All of these factors make it easier for your heart to pump blood throughout your body. These benefits are particularly beneficial to those who have pre-existing heart conditions, or partially clogged arteries, because they help reduce the risk of thrombotic heart attacks and strokes.

Benefits of Omega-3 Fatty Acids—
EPA and DHA

Research conducted by the Peking University People's Hospital in Beijing, China has shown that in patients who had suffered a previous heart attack, consumption of Omega-3 fatty acids reduced the rate of death from sudden cardiac death, a condition in which an abrupt radical change in heart rhythm brings on cardiac arrest. Finally, numerous studies suggest that an Omega-3-rich diet or supplementation with Omega-3s can lower blood pressure in people with hypertension.

Diabetes

Many diabetics exhibit reduced levels of "good" HDL—high density lipoprotein, cholesterol and triglycerides—both significant markers for the development of heart disease. Omega-3 fatty acids from fish oil can help lower triglycerides and apoproteins (markers of diabetes), and raise HDL. Research from the University of Malaga in Spain reveals that taking Omega-3s may increase the effectiveness of certain lipid-reducing statin drugs in diabetic patients. Since type 2 diabetes is one of the major risk factors for developing serious cardiovascular illness, this finding could help the development of more effective drugs for improving overall blood lipid levels.

Weight Control and Fitness

It is quite common for obese and overweight people to have a problem maintaining steady blood glucose levels due to insulin resistance. This causes insulin levels to spike and drop during the day, often resulting in extreme hunger, binge eating and the continuation of weight problems as well as disease markers like high cholesterol and arterial inflammation. However, it appears that essential fatty acids may stave off many of the otherwise deadly complications of obesity.

A study published in *The FASEB Journal* shows that two types of lipids the body manufactures after consuming essential fatty acids—protectins and resolvins—may protect the body against liver damage related to obesity and thus against future diabetes and other liver-related diseases. Overweight, diabetic mice that were fed a diet rich in Omega-3 fatty acids showed reduced inflammation and lower insulin resistance than control mice.

Benefits of Omega-3 Fatty Acids—
EPA and DHA

In addition, it appears that fish oil consumption actually improves the function of the cardiovascular system during exercise. A double-blind, placebo-controlled study carried out at the school of medicine at the University of Wollongong in New South Wales, Australia, revealed that athletes who were given daily fish oil supplements rich in EPA and DHA had reduced heart rates and lower oxygen consumption than control athletes. In short, essential fatty acids may increase the efficiency of the cardiovascular system during exercise.

Arthritis

Essential fatty acids have been shown in laboratory studies to reduce the body's levels of C-reactive protein, or CRP, a major marker of inflammation. In an analysis of 17 clinical trials that assessed the pain relieving effects of EPA and DHA supplementation in people with joint pain, researchers found that these fatty acids are an effective treatment for the pain associated with conditions like rheumatoid arthritis and inflammatory bowel disease, without the potentially dangerous side effects that can occur with non-steroidal anti-inflammatory drugs, or NSAIDs (acetaminophen, ibuprofen).

Osteoporosis

A Swedish study examined the blood fatty acid levels of 78 healthy young men while measuring the bone density in their hips, spines and entire bodies. The result: a clear correlation between each individual's serum Omega-3 levels and bone density. Just as interesting, higher ratios of Omega-6 to Omega-3 fatty acids correlated to the lower bone mass levels that can indicate a risk for future osteoporosis. In another trial, elderly men and women showed a similar link between Omega-3 levels and bone density, though this trial assessed essential fatty acid intake using dietary questionnaires rather than blood tests. Also, in a study of women over age 65 with osteoporosis, those given EPA and DHA supplements experienced significantly less bone loss (and many increased their bone density) over three years than those given a placebo.

Benefits of Omega-3 Fatty Acids—
EPA and DHA

Mental Illness

In a clinical study of patients who had been hospitalized for depression, the ratio of Omega-3 to Omega-6 fatty acids was found to be especially low. Another clinical study in which people with clinical depression ate Omega-3-rich fish several times a week for five years revealed a substantial reduction in major depression symptoms.

In a 2007 study of 55 adults carried out by Sarah Conklin, a neuroscientist at University of Pittsburgh Medical School, magnetic resonance imaging showed that the richer the person's diet was in DHA, the more brain tissue they had in three areas of the brain linked to mood: the amygdala, the hippocampus and the cingulate. So essential fatty acids may in fact help the brain produce more gray matter to regulate mood and emotion.

Essential fatty acids may also reduce the violent mood swings of bipolar disorder, or manic-depressive disease. A double-blind, placebo-controlled study carried out in 1999 looked at 30 patients with bipolar disorder and found that the patients who consumed Omega-3s had longer remissions between manic and depressive episodes and had less severe symptoms than patients in the control group who consumed olive oil.

Finally, preliminary evidence suggests that people with schizophrenia show improvement in symptoms when given omega-3 fatty acids. Researchers at the University of Sheffield in the UK have stated that EPA appears to yield the greatest benefits for patients with schizophrenia, typically in dosages of 2,000 to 4,000 mg per day.

Attention Deficit Hyperactivity Disorder (ADHD)

In a clinical study of nearly 100 boys, those with normal Omega-3 fatty acid levels had fewer problems with behavior and concentration than those with low levels. Additionally, animal studies have revealed that individuals deficient in Omega-3s often have lower levels of vital neurotransmitters like dopamine and serotonin, which are related to attention and motivation. Having essential fatty acids available as an adjunct therapy for ADHD provides children and their parents with healthful therapeutic options.

Benefits of Omega-3 Fatty Acids— EPA and DHA

Nutrient Connections

- CoQ10
- Arginine and citrulline (nitric oxide synthesis)
- Vitamin E

Interactions

Omega-3 fatty acids may decrease blood pressure and thin the blood. People taking prescription blood pressure medications and/or antico-agulants should consult with their health care provider.

Recommended Supplementation

- Maintenance of optimal health: 500 mg total Omega-3 per day
- Obesity, diabetes, cardiovascular dysfunction and other enhanced health concerns: 900 mg total Omega-3 (EPA: 647/DHA: 253) per day as a minimum

Chapter Thirteen
Glucosamine

Power Facts

✦ There are no food sources of glucosamine.

✦ The cartilage-to-cartilage interaction that occurs in our joints produces less friction with movement than ice on ice.

✦ Aspirin and NSAIDs (non-steroidal anti-inflammatories), which are commonly used to treat the symptoms of arthritis, may in fact inhibit the natural repair of joint tissue, thus leading to further damage.

✦ Our body's natural production of glucosamine slows with age.

Glucosamine has been marketed as a treatment and preventive supplement for osteoarthritis for many years. Solid science shows that this naturally occurring substance offers real benefits for joint health.

In a healthy state, the body makes glucosamine, a simple molecule composed of glucose and an *amine,* an organic derivative of ammonia. In the joints, its function is to stimulate the manufacture of key structural components of cartilage. Cartilage is one of the primary tissues that provide cushion and lubrication to the joints, especially in such areas as the knees, hips and spine. Unsurprisingly, these are the parts of the body where complaints of osteoarthritis pain are most frequent.

As some people age, they lose the ability to manufacture sufficient levels of glucosamine. The result is that cartilage loses its ability to act as a shock absorber. The weight bearing joints—the knees, hips, and joints of the hands—are those most often affected with osteoarthritis. In affected joints, cartilage destruction is followed by hardening and the formation of bone spurs in the joint margins, pain, deformity and limited range of motion. Supplemental glucosamine stimulates the manufacture of substances necessary for proper joint function and repair. Therefore, maintaining and replenishing cartilage is an important wellness issue, and it is here that glucosamine excels.

This led researchers in Europe to ask an important question; what would happen if individuals with osteoarthritis took glucosamine as a supplement? The European patent holder for glucosamine, Rottapharm, sponsored two three-year-long, placebo-controlled clinical trials of its brand of glucosamine sulfate using 100 patients or more, beginning in 2001. Both studies showed clear benefits, including reduced symptoms and healthier joints.

Uses

✦ **Osteoarthritis treatment.**
✦ **Osteoporosis treatment.**
✦ **Injury prevention and exercise performance enhancement.**

Benefits of Glucosamine

The primary use for glucosamine is the treatment of osteoarthritis, knee osteoarthritis in particular. Glucosamine is a safe, effective, natural alternative to aspirin and other NSAIDs. Clinical research indicates that NSAIDs may actually accelerate the progression of joint destruction, and also produce such symptoms as gastrointestinal upset and kidney damage.

This is why glucosamine provides such an effective alternative. The benefits of glucosamine in patients with osteoarthritis are likely the result of two important effects:

- Stimulation of the synthesis of *proteoglycans*, proteins associated with healthy joint tissues.

Benefits of Glucosamine

- Inhibiting the synthesis of substances that contribute to cartilage damage and cause the death of *articular chondrocytes*, cells that contribute to tissue repair.

Nutrient Connections

- Vitamin C (supports collagen formation)
- Vitamin E
- Vitamins A, B6, Zinc, Copper and Boron

Interactions

Individuals taking diuretic medications may need to increase their glucosamine intake for maximum effectiveness.

Recommended Supplementation

- 1,500 mg per day
- Obese individuals may require more glucosamine; 20 mg per kilogram of body weight is recommended.

Chapter Fourteen
Green Tea

Power Facts

✦ Archeological evidence suggests that people consumed tea leaves steeped in boiling water as many as 5,000 years ago.

✦ The primary antioxidant in green tea (EGCG) is 100 times more potent than vitamins C and E.

✦ One cup of green tea (delivering 10-40 mg of antioxidant polyphenols) has antioxidant effects greater than a serving of broccoli, spinach or carrots.

✦ Green tea is tremendously beneficial.

✦ Green tea has the highest polyphenol content, while black tea has roughly two to three times the caffeine content of green tea.

Drinking tea has for centuries been associated with health and wellness, as well as for the meditative, almost Zen quality of the tea drinking experience, especially when in the context of something like a Japanese tea ceremony. However, a growing collection of clinical research is showing that green tea as a phytochemical and nutrient has many powerful qualities that are beneficial to health.

Archeological evidence suggests that tea has been consumed for almost 5,000 years. Green tea is still used as a traditional medicine in India, China, Japan, and

Thailand to aid in healthcare concerns ranging from controlling bleeding and healing wounds to regulating blood sugar and promoting healthy digestion.

Green tea and black tea are made from the same plant, *Camellia sinensis*. However, in processing green tea, the leaves are left largely unaltered, so they retain their green color and their vital nutrients remain unoxidized. This is why even though all teas, including white and oolong varieties, contain the powerful antioxidants EGCG, (epigallocatechin gallate), catechins and flavonoids, green tea, which is considered a "true tea," contains them at their highest levels. It also contains other beneficial molecules such as amino acids and polyphenols that may offer their own considerable health advantages.

Uses

+ Obesity and weight management.
+ Immune support and general vitality.
+ Metabolic syndrome and type 2 diabetes treatment.
+ Treatment of cardiovascular dysfunction.
+ Cancer prevention.

Benefits of Green Tea

Green tea offers powerful free-radical scavenging properties, especially in conditions of high oxidative stress (diabetes, metabolic syndrome, cardiovascular dysfunction). It promotes healthy metabolic function and supports the maintenance of a healthy body weight, and helps maintain healthful cholesterol and triglyceride levels. It also elevates levels of the "good" HDL cholesterol, which protects against coronary artery disease.

Over the last few decades, green tea has been the subject of many scientific and medical studies to determine the extent of its health benefits. Some evidence suggests that regular green tea drinkers are at lower risk for heart disease and certain types of cancer. A 2006 study published in the *Journal of the American Medical Association* concluded that, "Green tea consumption is associated with reduced mortality due to all causes and due to cardiovascular disease but not with reduced mortality due to cancer." The study, conducted by the Tohoku University School of Public Policy in Japan, followed 40,530 healthy Japanese adults for up to 11 years, monitoring for death from all causes and for up to seven years for death from a specific cause, such as heart disease. The study found that the adults who consumed five or more cups of green tea per day had a 16% lower risk of mortality from all causes—and a 26% lower risk of cardiovascular disease than those who drank less than one cup per day.

Then, in May 2006, a Yale University School of Medicine team performed its own meta-analysis of more than 100 green tea studies and trials. Their results indicated an "Asian paradox:" lower rates of heart disease and cancer in Asians despite high rates of cigarette smoking. Their theory suggested that the 1.2 liters of green tea consumed per day by the average Asian delivered a protective effect via its potent antioxidants and other compounds, and that this protective effect shielded drinkers from cardiovascular damage in part by keeping blood platelets from sticking together to form dangerous clots and reducing the buildup of artery-clogging LDL cholesterol.

Cardiovascular Dysfunction and Atherosclerosis

Population-based clinical studies (studies that follow large groups of people for an extended period) indicate that the antioxidant properties of green tea may help prevent atherosclerosis, particularly coronary artery disease.

High Cholesterol

Research shows that green tea lowers total cholesterol and raises HDL ("good") cholesterol in both animals and people. One population-based clinical study found that men who drink green tea are more likely to have lower total cholesterol than those who do not. Results from one animal study suggest that polyphenols in green tea may block the intestinal absorption of cholesterol and promote its excretion from the body. In another small study of male smokers, researchers found that green tea significantly reduced blood levels of harmful LDL cholesterol.

Cancer

Several population-based clinical studies have shown that green tea helps protect against cancer. For example, cancer rates tend to be low in countries such as

Japan where people regularly consume green tea. Researchers also believe that polyphenols help kill cancerous cells and stop their progression.

In one study of 472 women with various stages of breast cancer, researchers found that women who consumed the most green tea experienced the least spreading of cancer. They also found that women with early stages of the disease who drank at least five cups of tea every day before being diagnosed with cancer were less likely to suffer recurrences of the disease after completion of treatment.

In a clinical study conducted on ovarian cancer patients in China, researchers found that women who drank at least one cup of green tea per day survived longer with the disease than those who didn't drink green tea. In fact, those who drank the most tea lived the longest.

Liver Disease

Population-based clinical studies have shown that men who drink more than 10 cups of green tea per day are less likely to develop disorders of the liver. Green tea also seems to protect the liver from the damaging effects of toxic substances such as alcohol.

Weight Loss

Clinical studies suggest that green tea extract may boost metabolism and help burn fat. One study confirmed that the combination of green tea and caffeine improved weight loss and maintenance in overweight and moderately obese individuals.

An Indiana trial looked at 107 overweight or obese adults who consumed a drink containing green tea catechins versus adults who consumed a beverage containing only caffeine and found that the green tea catechins seemed to enhance the effects of moderate exercise on weight loss, abdominal fat loss, and reduction of triglycerides. A similar study performed in Japan and published in the *Journal of Nutrition* showed similar results: people who consumed high levels of catechins had lower abdominal fat levels and lost more overall body weight than the control group.

Cognitive Function

A 2009 Oxford University study revealed that the consumption of flavonoids, one of the potent antioxidants found in green tea, dramatically improved cognition on tests in people age 70 to 74, an indication that perhaps green tea could be part of a program to prevent or delay age-related dementia and loss of cognitive function.

Nutrient Connections

- Vitamins C and E
- Pomegranate
- Chromium picolinate

Interactions

None

Recommended Supplementation

- For general health promotion, two to three cups of green tea per day (for a total of 240 to 320 mg of polyphenols)
- 100 to 750 mg per day of standardized green tea extract (98% polyphenols and 45% EGCG) is recommended. Caffeine-free products are available and recommended if you prefer.

Chapter Fifteen
Pomegranate

The humble pomegranate, best known for its sticky, staining seeds, has become another of our nutritional superstars. This exotic fruit turns out to be a powerhouse of antioxidants with significant health promoting benefits.

The pomegranate (*Punica granatum*) is a fruit-bearing small tree that grows primarily in Iran, India, Afghanistan, Algeria, Armenia, Pakistan, Syria, Turkey, parts of southeast Asia and Malaysia, and tropical Africa, and is now cultivated in California and Arizona. One of the earliest cultivated fruits, the pomegranate has been part of popular lore and wellness regimens for thousands of years and has been associated with health and rebirth by numerous cultures.

Benefits of Pomegranate

Several studies indicate that pomegranate juice may prevent cartilage deterioration and thus prevent the progress of osteoarthritis. It also prevents plaque from building up in the arteries and may reverse previous plaque buildup, arresting the development of coronary artery disease. It reduces undesirable LDL cholesterol levels while increasing levels of HDL cholesterol. Finally, one study showed that drinking 1.7 ounces of pomegranate juice per day lowered systolic blood pressure by as much as 5%.

Cholesterol

The tannins in pomegranate juice appear to reduce several heart disease risk factors, including the oxidation of "bad" cholesterol.

A pilot study on 19 patients with atherosclerosis demonstrated a reduction in arterial plaque growth. After one year, arterial plaque decreased 30% for those patients who consumed pomegranate juice daily, compared to a 9% worsening for patients who drank a placebo.

Blood Pressure

It has been shown to reduce blood pressure by inhibiting angiotensin-converting enzyme, or ACE, the molecule that causes vessels to constrict and is also inhibited by prescription medications like Benazepril.

Cardiovascular Dysfunction

In a 2005 study published in the *American Journal of Cardiology*, researchers studied a total of 45 patients with coronary heart disease who had reduced blood flow to the heart. The results showed improved blood flow to the heart in patients drinking eight ounces of daily pomegranate juice for three months. Patients drinking pomegranate juice experienced a 17% improvement in blood flow, compared to a worsening of 18% in patients drinking a placebo.

Cancer

A preliminary study published by *The American Association for Cancer Research* found hopeful results for prostate health. The UCLA study followed 46 men previously treated for prostate cancer either with surgery or radiation.

Dr. Ignarro's Published Research on Pomegranate

Pomegranate juice protects nitric oxide against oxidative destruction and enhances the biological actions of nitric oxide. Ignarro LJ, Byrns RE, Sumi D, de Nigris F, Napoli C. Nitric Oxide 15(2): 93-102, 2006.

Pomegranate contains antioxidants capable of markedly protecting Nitric Oxide against free radical destruction, while augmenting certain biological actions of nitric oxide such as inhibition of vascular smooth muscle cell proliferation. These research observations support the conclusions that pomegranate possesses potent antioxidant activity that is associated with anti-atherosclerotic effects in humans.

Pomegranate juice helps promote healthy coronary endothelial cells by enhancing nitric oxide. de Nigris F, Williams-Ignarro S, Botti C, Sica V, Ignarro LJ, and Napoli C. Nitric Oxide. 15(3):259-63, 2006.

By using pomegranate juice as a therapeutic intervention, Dr. Ignarro and his fellow researchers demonstrated that it is possible to attenuate the development of vascular damage associated with decreased nitric oxide activity. Antioxidant protection by pomegranate helps to decrease the production and release of free radicals in the vascular wall and improves the biologic and antioxidant activity of nitric oxide.

Benefits of Pomegranate

After drinking eight ounces of pomegranate juice daily for two years, these research subjects experienced significantly slower PSA (prostate specific antigen) doubling times: from 15 months at the beginning of the study to 54 months at the end. PSA is a biomarker for prostate cancer, and slower PSA doubling time may indicate slower disease progression.

Açai: Another Great Super Fruit

Açai (ah-sah-EE) is the small, round, black-purple fruit of a South American palm that has become the latest sensation in the realm of super fruit. The reason for its popularity is simple: it contains several different antioxidant compounds beneficial to health, including oleic acid, palmitic acid, linoleic acid, and polyphenols.

Originally a foodstuff in traditional rainforest cultures, açai has become an important supplement. It contains beta-sitosterol, a plant sterol that competes with dietary cholesterol for absorption, and so may reduce blood cholesterol levels. A recent study found that 19 amino acids can be found in açai, with especially high levels of aspartic acid and glutamic acid. In addition, the dense pigmentation of açai has led scientists to conduct several experimental studies of its anthocyanins, a group of polyphenols that gives the deep color to berries.

Benefits

A recent study demonstrated that açai contains several flavonoid compounds that are beneficial. Proanthocyanidins, another group of polyphenol compounds high in antioxidant value, are abundant in the pulp and skin of the fruit. Açai turns out to be effective at suppressing superoxide, thought to be the initial producer of more potent reactive oxygen species, the compounds that attack cells. This makes it a potent antioxidant and a powerful first line of defense against cell damage.

Erectile Dysfunction

A pilot study released in the *International Journal of Impotence Research* examined 61 male subjects with mild to moderate erectile dysfunction. Compared to research subjects taking a placebo, those men drinking eight ounces of pomegranate juice daily for four weeks were 50% more likely to experience improved erections.

Nutrient Connections

- Arginine, citrulline
- Vitamin C, Alpha lipoic acid

Interactions

A study from the Tufts University School of Medicine published in the *Journal of Clinical Pharmacology* finds that pomegranate juice does not interact with oral or intravenous medication, contrary to previous information. Earlier studies erroneously suggested that, like grapefruit juice, pomegranate juice may interfere with the metabolism of drugs by inhibiting an enzyme that allows the body to transform and eliminate a drug.

Recommended Supplementation

- Juice: 8 to 16 ounces of 100% pomegranate juice per day
- Supplement: Natural pomegranate polyphenol extract (standardized to 30% punicalagins) 1,000 mg per day

Chapter Sixteen

Vitamin D

Power Facts

✦ Vitamin D deficiency is a major public health problem, impacting people of all ages including both the young and the elderly.

✦ As many as half of older adults in the United States with hip fractures could have insufficient Vitamin D levels.

✦ Two studies have examined actual vitamin D levels in obese subjects. One found dramatically lower levels. A South Carolina study found all of the obese subjects had levels below 2.2 ng/ml (deficient) while all of the non-obese subjects had levels above 8 ng/ml (normal).

✦ Researchers found that 36% of young medical students and hospital residents— people who work long hours and rarely see the light of day—were Vitamin D insufficient at the end of winter.

It is estimated that one billion people around the world are Vitamin D deficient. Depending on your skin type, the latitude where you live (and thus the sun's intensity) the cloud cover, any sunscreen or clothing you are wearing and other factors, it takes 5-30 minutes of unprotected sun exposure twice per week to synthesize the necessary Vitamin D from precursor chemicals present in the skin. UV radiation from the sun is a known carcinogen and you should limit your exposure, but avoiding sunlight altogether is equally unhealthy. Vitamin D has been in the news commonly in recent years and for good reason: it appears to offer an astonishing range of potent health benefits.

Vitamin D is a group of fat soluble pro-hormones, the two major forms being D2 (ergocalciferol) and D3 (cholecalciferol). It is consumed in foods that either contain it naturally or are fortified with it, and your skin manufactures it when exposed to sunlight.

Vitamin D is not naturally present in significant quantities in many foods. Salmon, tuna, mackerel and fish liver oils are among the best sources, while beef liver, cheese, and egg yolks provide small amounts. But in general, supplementation or regular sun exposure is necessary to avoid deficiency. Deficiency can also occur due to diseases that prevent Vitamin D absorption. Vitamin D deficiency has been linked to colon cancer, as well as an increased susceptibility to high blood pressure, tuberculosis, multiple sclerosis, mental illness, and autoimmune diseases.

Our need for Vitamin D increases with age, even as the ability of the skin to manufacture and the kidneys to synthesize it both decrease. These factors increase the importance of Vitamin D supplementation in the elderly.

Uses

+ Offers protective effects against several types of cancer.
+ Promotes bone mineralization and formation.
+ Reduces risk of cardiovascular dysfunction and heart attacks.
+ Supports healthy immune system activity and reducing infections.

Benefits of Vitamin D

Osteoporosis

Vitamin D helps the body absorb and use calcium, making it a factor in the development and maintenance of bone mass. Healthy bone is a dynamic system that is constantly being replaced, so sufficient levels of Vitamin D are needed to make the process of mineralization optimal. Few studies on the effect of supplementation on osteoporosis have separated calcium benefits from Vitamin D benefits, but as we stated in the chapter on the osteoporosis-osteoarthritis syndrome, it is becoming clearer that Vitamin D deficiency is a major contributing factor to the development of a brittle, fracture-prone skeletal system.

Cancer and Immune Health

Vitamin D appears to offer a protective effect against several types of cancer. A study done at the International Epidemiology Institute in Rockville, Maryland, revealed that patients with higher levels of Vitamin D intake exhibited the lowest levels of colon cancer, suggesting a possible protective effect. A study from the University of Edinburgh in Scotland revealed the same correlation between high levels of Vitamin D and reduced colon cancer risk. Other research has shown that men with the highest Vitamin D levels had the lowest risk of advanced colon cancer.

Additional research published in the *Journal of the National Cancer Institute* suggests that high Vitamin D levels may lower the risk of oral and esophageal cancers, pancreatic cancer, and leukemia. Increased Vitamin D intake may cut the risk of prostate, breast, and ovarian cancers, according to a 2006 review of research findings on the links between Vitamin D and cancer published in the *American Journal of Public Health.*

Cardiovascular Disease

Researchers at Harvard Medical School reported that Vitamin D deficiency is associated with an increase in high blood pressure and cardiovascular risks. For more than 1,700 patients with an average age of 59, they monitored Vitamin D levels, blood pressure and other cardiovascular risk factors for five years. The conclusion: people with low levels of Vitamin D had a 62% higher risk of cardiovascular disease or heart attack than those with normal Vitamin D levels. Another Harvard study found the same results in young women.

A 2009 Johns Hopkins study of teenagers and Vitamin D levels is an example of the strong correlation between Vitamin D levels and disease risk. In the study, teens with the lowest levels of Vitamin D in their blood had a 400% increase in their risk of developing the metabolic syndrome, a 250% higher risk of having dangerously high blood sugar levels, and more than double the risk of high blood pressure than teens with the highest Vitamin D levels. All are factors for developing cardiovascular disease later in life.

Obesity

A Medical College of Georgia study conducted in 2009 revealed that of 650 teens aged 14 to 19 studied, those with the highest serum levels of Vitamin D had the lowest levels of overall body fat as well as the lowest levels of visceral fat, the abdominal fat linked to high cholesterol and heart disease. In addition, several other recent studies have established a firm link between seasonal Vitamin D levels (which are based on sun exposure and the duration of the day) and obesity.

Cognitive Health

Research carried out by the Peninsula Medical School in Exeter, the University of Cambridge, and the University of Michigan shows a strong inverse relationship between Vitamin D levels and age-related cognitive decline. The study looked at more than 2,000 individuals over age 64 and found that those who performed poorly on tests of memory, attention and orientation in time and space were deficient in Vitamin D. This result supports a prior study that found that older patients with some form of dementia had lower blood levels of Vitamin D than their fellow subjects with higher or near-normal Vitamin D levels.

Arthritis

Work done at Johannes Gutenberg University of Mainz in Germany found that 84.7% of men and women undergoing total hip or knee replacement due to disability caused by osteoarthritis had a Vitamin D deficiency, bolstering the link between low bone density (a frequent result of a Vitamin D deficiency) and osteoarthritis.

An even stronger connection between Vitamin D and arthritis comes from the Iowa Women's Health Study, which followed almost 30,000 women, aged 55 to 69, for 11 years. During the trial, 152 of the women developed rheumatoid arthritis. The investigators found that women whose diets were highest in Vitamin D had the lowest incidence of rheumatoid arthritis.

Infections

Researchers from the University of Colorado, Denver have found that Vitamin D offers significant protection against common diseases like colds and flu. A study of about 19,000 adults and adolescents found that people with the lowest average levels of Vitamin D in their blood were about 40% more likely to have had a recent respiratory infection, compared to those without a Vitamin D deficiency.

The findings, published in *Archives of Internal Medicine*, suggest that Vitamin D may somehow support the immune system in the fight against common viral maladies. This might also explain the findings of a few years ago that revealed that colds and flu do not spread as readily in warm, humid, tropical climates—regions where the earth's orientation means more sun exposure for the population.

Overall Death Rate

A Johns Hopkins study in early 2009 showed that high Vitamin D levels reduce overall mortality from any health-related cause by 26% over a period of eight years. So your risk of dying from heart disease, cancer, stroke, diabetes, kidney failure, and other major killers may be reduced simply by adding more of the "sunshine Vitamin" to your diet.

Nutrient Connections

- Calcium
- Magnesium
- Vitamin B6
- Folic acid
- Vitamin B12

Interactions

The drugs cholestryramine, dilantin and phenobarbital interfere with the absorption and/or metabolism of Vitamin D.

Recommended Supplementation

Vitamin D3: 2,000 IU to 5,000 IU per day. Research evidence may extend the dosage of Vitamin D3 to 10,000 IU per day for certain health conditions.

Chapter Seventeen

Simple Health Value

In summary, the philosophy behind *Health Is Wealth* is a simple and positive one: you have control over your health and longevity. This idea is borne out by, among many other studies, the 25-year MacArthur Study of Successful Aging, which found that longevity is 70% based on lifestyle decisions, 25% based on genetics, and 5% based on luck. So, unless you are in the tiny minority who inherited a genetic disease from your parents, you are not a prisoner of your hereditary health status. Even if your father and grandfather died from heart attacks by age 60, that does not condemn you to the same fate. It elevates your risk, but such information represents your *potential* health outcome, not fate. You can control how your genes express themselves and how your body changes over time through the lifestyle choices you make.

It's no secret that in this book, we promote supplementation as one of those positive lifestyle changes. Taking key Power Nutrients via dietary supplements is such a simple, cost-effective and empowering way to combat Nutrient Depletion Syndrome that it's not surprising that, according to the Council for Responsible Nutrition, 68% of Americans say they take dietary supplements over the course of a year. The question is, are they taking the right combination of supplements for their wellness and health risk? That is a question you and a trained healthcare professional should answer together. If you're working right now with a doctor or other care provider who disagrees with the concept of nutritional supplementation as a path toward greater wellness, then it's time to find a health professional with a more progressive view.

As we hope we have demonstrated, a vast repository of solid science supports the idea that supplementation can overcome nutritional deficiencies caused by our modern diet, farming and food production methods and our stressful lifestyles. As you consider what we have said in this book and look at starting your own supplementation plan or revising your current program, we recommend the following steps:

1. Do your own research. Doctors and dieticians don't know everything, and sometimes some timely research will bring to light facts or discoveries that your healthcare provider wasn't aware of.
2. Examine your diet. Are you getting enough of some nutrients now through what you eat? How can you improve your diet?
3. Talk to your physician about any health conditions you may have now or any risk factors you have for future disease. This will inform the choices and dosages of supplements you take.
4. Look at any medications you currently take and discuss possible side effects. Many medications block or inhibit the actions of nutrients within the body. If you don't consider that, you're flying blind.
5. Be careful of hype. A lot of unqualified people make a lot of outlandish claims about "natural" supplements. Be sure there is solid scientific evidence to support the claims.

Keep in mind that unless you are taking a supplement to address a specific health condition, such as type 2 diabetes, you may not feel very different right away, even after taking a custom-designed cocktail of Power Nutrients. This is because our wellness strategy is designed to promote long-term healing and the optimal function of your body's systems, from energy metabolism and blood sugar control to brain function and cardiovascular health. You may not get a sudden buzz of energy or feel like a million dollars overnight. That's not the point of the *Health Is Wealth* philosophy. It's designed to bring you improved wellness and a sense of well-being over time, so while you might not notice a dramatic overnight shift in your energy, over a year or more you will probably find yourself feeling better, looking better and most importantly, getting better results when you have your annual physical exam.

Recession-Proof Health

Over the time we have been working on this book, we have watched the global economy fall farther and farther into a state of near-collapse. This, of course, not only affects people's homes, jobs and retirements, but also their health, as millions lose healthcare benefits after being laid off from work and millions more forego doctor visits and other medical attention because they simply cannot afford it. We are in the middle of a healthcare crisis of unprecedented proportions.

However, as we've already discussed, you can gain some control over your healthcare costs in a time of economic chaos by being proactive. The *Health Is Wealth* strategy is based on taking charge of your wellness before a serious health problem arises—about making yourself as "disease-proof" as possible. By doing so, you will prevent many of the health conditions that force people with scant financial resources to either spend money they don't have on medical care or go without and risk developing a health crisis.

In the same vein, we promote the concept of Simple Health Value, a companion to our Power Nutrient supplementation approach. You see, ensuring maximal wellness for years and decades to come is about your comprehensive lifestyle choices; nothing exists in isolation in the body. So you cannot embark on a Power Nutrient supplement regimen while refusing to exercise, eating junk food, smoking and exposing yourself to daily stress. No nutrient—not Vitamin D, not Omega-3 fatty acids, not antioxidants—is powerful enough to counteract a poor lifestyle. So if you truly want to optimize your well-being and give yourself the best odds possible of passing through your 60s, 70s and beyond without experiencing the debilitating health problems of so many Americans, you must change *everything* about how you live—how you eat, move, sleep, play and deal with the pressures of life. Fortunately, there is a way to do this that does not feel like you're being sent to boot camp. And it costs very little, which is more important than ever today.

Simple Health Value

The concept of Simple Health Value is built on five basic principles that perfectly complement the Power Nutrient program we've discussed. They are:

1. Drink more water.
2. Eat fresh food.
3. Move daily.
4. Get more rest.
5. Breathe deeply every day.

That's it. What makes the Simple Health Value approach so effective for people of all backgrounds and all health levels is this: *it doesn't take anything away.* That's revolutionary. We're not telling you that you've got to give up a group of foods, stop drinking soda and so on. Would your health improve if you quit eating fast food burgers in favor of salads? Probably. But one of the most certain ways to fail at counseling people in making important lifestyle changes is to lecture and wag your finger at them. No one likes to be told all the things they're doing wrong. It's a sure path to resentment and refusal to cooperate, even when something is in their best interest.

So Simple Health Value takes the opposite approach: adding good health value to your daily life. We don't ask you to take anything away, just to add good things. Over time, as adding beneficial choices to your daily routine makes you feel and look healthier, you may decide on your own to do away with poor habits or unhealthy foods, but then it will be your decision. That's the only way real lifestyle change lasts: when you choose it for yourself because it becomes a priority. So as you contemplate how to use the nutrient information we have shared with you, also make the five components of Simple Health Value part of your overall "living to 100" plan.

1. Drink more water. Water is still the best liquid you can put into your body. Aside from fending off dehydration, drinking water has at least two strong, proven benefits. First, if you drink before you eat a meal, you will feel fuller and eat less, which makes water a great tool for losing and maintaining weight. The second benefit also relates to body weight: drinking cold water increases the body's metabolic rate as more energy is used to bring the water to body temperature. Drinking enough water also keeps your kidneys flushed out and working properly, so while the main priority is to stay hydrated, drinking clear, cool water does offer some nice bonuses.

2. Eat fresh food. This means consuming more fresh fruits and vegetables daily. Simple Health Value is not about cutting certain foods out of your diet, but adding a snack of baby carrots while you're at your desk, dumping some blueberries on top of your morning cereal, or eating crisp red grapes as a snack when you're done working out. The overall plan here is to introduce as much whole, unprocessed food into your body as possible by "shopping the perimeter" of the grocery store—steering clear of the central aisles where the processed food is and going for fresh produce, nuts, seeds, nonfat dairy, fish, and poultry.

Organic is better, and grown in your own garden is best, but whatever the source, the goal should be to add 4 to 6 servings of fruit and/or vegetables to your diet every day, and the more variety the better. By eating in this way, you'll be doing more than getting vital Power Nutrients. You'll also be getting the fiber and other additional components of whole food that help nutrients work better, as well as phytochemicals and other compounds we don't fully understand yet.

3. Move daily. Let's do the math on getting a little more exercise each day. First of all, weight loss over the short and long term comes down to two factors—eat less and move more. A study released in 2009 confirmed what nutrition and weight loss experts have said for years: it's about calories, not the type of food you eat. Now, the type of food affects other aspects of health such as cholesterol and blood sugar, but if you're trying to get down to a healthy body weight, a calorie is a calorie.

A calorie is simply a unit of heat energy, the amount of heat needed to raise one cubic centimeter of water by one degree Celsius. Eating food containing enough energy to produce 3,500 calories will produce one pound of stored body fat if your body does not expend those calories as energy. So if you want to lose a pound of fat, you've got to burn 3,500 more calories than you take in. Let's say that you weigh 250 pounds and hate exercise but you want to lose weight. You don't change your diet at all, but you start walking to and from work each day, a round-trip distance of two miles. If you walked at an average pace of three mph, you would burn about 265 extra calories per day.

That means that if you walked five days per week to and from your workplace and changed *nothing else* about your lifestyle, you would lose about 19 pounds in the next year. If you made no other changes at all, in three years this simple strategy of adding a little movement to your day's routine would get you down to 200 pounds or perhaps even 190 (you might plateau as you got closer to 200 and lose less weight). And because the weight loss was gradual and came with a lifestyle change, you would likely keep the weight off, as well as slashing your risk for diabetes, heart disease and cancer.

So, how does the idea of moving your body a little more each day sound now? Do you think you could walk two miles a day, take the stairs instead of the elevator or do your own gardening if it meant a dramatic improvement in your health?

4. Get more rest. This isn't just about sleep, although it could be since according to the National Sleep Foundation 70 million Americans suffer from some sort of sleep disorder. We're also talking about rest, that mental downtime in which we are awake but resting our minds and senses—not answering the cell phone or checking e-mail. Rest and sleep are enormously important mechanisms to cope with stress, and as we've discussed, intimately related to the development of clinical depression.

The Simple Health Value prescription for rest is easy: make downtime and sleep priorities. Too often in our culture we make sleeplessness heroic, as though depriving ourselves of that which replenishes our bodies and minds is something to be proud of. It isn't. It's a sure way to hamper mental performance and exacerbate the long-term effects of stress hormones. Instead of celebrating insomnia, we recommend creating your own sleep rituals, in which sleep is something sacred, with its own space and its own pre-sleep routine. As for rest, simply carve out time in your day for 15 minutes of quiet meditation, a walk in nature, or just daydreaming. All these activities allow the brain to rest and replenish neurochemicals and can increase well-being and concentration—and they certainly don't hurt your blood pressure, either.

5. Breathe deeply every day. Quick, how are you breathing right now? We're all unaware of our breathing at any particular time, but most of us breathe shallow most of the day. Shallow breathing reduces the body's oxygen levels, can reduce energy levels and increases the stress response. When you breathe fast and shallow, your body interprets this to mean that something stressful is happening, and the fight-or-flight response kicks in. This can mean the release of cortisol and other powerful hormones that over time drive up blood pressure, damage arteries and do the harm that we've talked about.

Conscious deep breathing is one of the best ways to reduce the effects of stress and bring on an immediate feeling of well-being. Try it now and you'll see. Breathing is the only autonomic nervous function over which we can exercise conscious control, and doing so can have a powerful relaxing effect on the body. When breathing slows and deepens, the body's stress response backs down. Heart rate and blood pressure drop. Everything relaxes. This is why products designed to reduce blood pressure by teaching patients to breathe deeply in patterns have been approved by the FDA; they work.

A Potent Strategy

Imagine if you combined the five Simple Health Value steps with a daily Power Nutrient supplementation plan. You would be doing virtually everything possible to correct any nutrient deficiencies, optimize your current health and prevent disease down the line. You would also give yourself the best odds for preventing ruinous healthcare costs and living a long, vital life. And all this requires is a choice on your part.

We've given you the information. We've given you the justification and the facts and the best advice we can give. The rest is up to you. Health really is wealth in more ways than just financial, and whatever choices you make, we wish you riches.

Endnotes

Chapter 4

Kenchaiah, Satish M.D., Evans, Jane C. D.Sc., Levy, Daniel M.D., Wilson, Peter W.F. M.D., Benjamin, Emelia J. M.D., Larson, Martin G. S.D., Kannel, William B. M.D., M.P.H., and Vasan, Ramachandran S. M.D. Obesity and the Risk of Heart Failure *New England Journal of Medicine* Volume 347:305-313, August 1, 2002, Number 5.

Natori, Shunsuke, Lai, Shenghan, Finn, J. Paul, Gomes, Antoinette S., Hundley, W. Gregory, Jerosch-Herold, Michael, Pearson, Gregory, Sinha, Shantanu, Arai, Andrew, Lima, Joao A. C. and Bluemke, David A. Cardiovascular Function in Multi-Ethnic Study of Atherosclerosis: Normal Values by Age, Sex, and Ethnicity. *American Journal of Roentgenology* 2006; 186:S357-S365.

Selvin, Elizabeth , Coresh, Josef, Golden, Sherita H., Brancati, Frederick L., Folsom, Aaron R. and Steffes, Michael W. High Blood Sugar Levels a Risk Factor for Heart Disease Diabetics and Non-Diabetics at Increased Risk, *John Hopkins/Bloomberg School of Public Health Dept. of Epidemiology* September 13, 2005.

Furberg, Curt D. Treatment of Hypertension: A Failing Report Card. *American Journal of Hypertension* (2009); 22, 1, 1–2.

Chapter 5

National Center for Research Resources (NCRR). Study of Depression, Peptides, and Steroids in Cushing's Syndrome. *ClinicalTrials*.gov Identifier NCT00004334.

Mezzich, J.E., Peralta, V., Cuesta, M.J. Sleeplessness and Paranoid Thinking. *World Psychiatry. Official Journal of the WPA* Volume 6, Number 2, June 2007.

Tasali, Esra and Penev, Plamen (University of Chicago) and Spiegel, Karine (Universite Libre de Bruxelles, Belgium). The National Institutes of Health, the European Sleep Research Society, the Belgian Fonds de la Recherche Scientifique Medicale, the University of Chicago Diabetes Research and Training Grant and the University of Chicago Clinical Research Center funded this study. Sleep loss boosts appetite, may encourage weight gain. December 6, 2004.

Ohayon, Maurice M., and Roth, Thomas. Place of chronic insomnia in the course of depressive and anxiety disorders. *Journal of Psychiatric Research* 2003; Vol. 37: pages 9-15.

Docherty, John. Chromium picolinate may reduce depression symptoms. *Nutraingredients-usa.com* 03-Jun-2004.

Naftalin, Richard, Afzal, Iram, Cunningham, Philip, Ross, Clare, Salleh, Naguib and Milligan, Staurt. Interactions of testosterone, androstenedione, green tea catechins and the anti-androgen Flutamide with the external glucose binding site of the human glucose transporter, *GLUT1*. University of College London (2003), J Physiol 547P, C133.

Chapter 6

Nevitt, Michael C. Department of Epidemiology and Biostatistics, University of California, San Francisco. Obesity Outcomes in Disease Management: Clinical Outcomes for Osteoarthritis, *Obesity Research* (2002) 10, 33S–37S.

Hart, D, Spector, T, Egger, P, Coggon, D and Cooper, C. Defining osteoarthritis of the hand for epidemiological studies: the Chingford Study. *Ann Rheum Dis* 1994 April; 53(4): 220–223.

Ragovin, Helene. The Possible Adventures of Super D. Tufts University Vitamin Research Department 2009. *Tufts Nutrition* Fall 2008.

Glowacki, Julie PhD, Hurwitz, Shelley PhD, Thornhill, Thomas S. MD, Kelly, Michael BA and LeBoff , Meryl S. MD. Osteoporosis and Vitamin-D Deficiency Among Postmenopausal Women with Osteoarthritis Undergoing Total Hip Arthroplasty. *The Journal of Bone and Joint Surgery* (American) 85:2371-2377 (2003).

McAlindon, Timothy E. DM; Felson, David T. MD; Zhang, Yuqing DSc; Hannan, Marian T. DSc; Aliabadi, Piran MD; Weissman, Barbara MD; Rush, David MD; Wilson, Peter W.F. MD; and Jacques, Paul ScD. Relation of Dietary Intake and Serum Levels of Vitamin D to Progression of Osteoarthritis of the Knee among Participants in the Framingham Study. *Annals of Internal Medicine* 1 September 1996 Volume 125 Number 5.

Dr. James Dowd. *The Vitamin D Cure.* New Jersey: Wiley Publications, 2009

Chapter 7

Berkson, Burton M. MD, MS, PhD. Alpha Lipoic Acid and Liver Disease. *Douglas Laboratories NutriNews* Vol 4, No.2, 1996.

Hager K, Marahrens A, Kenklies M, Riederer P, Munch G. Alpha-Lipoic Acid as a New Treatment Option for Azheimer Type Dementia. *Arch Gerontol Geriatr* 2001 Jun; 32 (3): 275-282.

Larsen, Hans R. MSc ChE. Alpha-Lipoic Acid: The Universal Antioxidant. *International Health News* ISSN 1203-1933.

Campochiaro, Peter et al. Scientists slow vision loss with vitamin E, alpha-lipoic acid and other antioxidant chemicals. *Medical Research News* 24. July 2006 06:56.

Chapter 8

Dawson, Beryl APD; Favaloro, Emmanuel J. PhD. High Rate of Deficiency in the Amino Acids Tryptophan and Histidine in People with Wounds: Implication for Nutrient Targeting in Wound Management-A Pilot Study. *Advances in Skin & Wound Care* February 2009 - Volume 22 - Issue 2 - pp 79-82.

Zhang ,Cheng, Gao, Kim Sung-Jin. Taurine Induces Anti-Anxiety by Activating Strychnine-Sensitive Glycine Receptor in vivo. *Annals of Nutrition and Metabolism* Vol. 51, No. 4, 2007.

Jobgen, Wenjuan, Meininger, Cynthia J., Jobgen, Scott C., Li, Peng, Lee, Mi-Jeong, Smith, Stephen B., Spencer, Thomas E., Fried, Susan K. and Wu, Guoyao. Dietary L-Arginine Supplementation Reduces White Fat Gain and Enhances Skeletal Muscle and Brown Fat Masses in Diet-Induced Obese Rats1–3. *Journal of Nutrition* Vol. 139, No. 2, 230-237, February 2009.

Chapter 9

Erlund, Iris, Koli, Raika, Alfthan, Georg, Marniemi, Jukka, Puukka, Pauli, Mustonen, Pirjo, Mattila, Pirjo and Jula, Antti. Favorable effects of berry consumption on platelet function, blood pressure, and HDL cholesterol. *American Journal of Clinical Nutrition* Vol. 87, No. 2, 323-331, February 2008.

Hana, Sung Nim, Meydania, Mohsen, Wua, Dayong, Benderb, Bradley S., Smitha, Donald E., Viñac, José, Caod, Guohua, Priora, Ronald L. and Meydania, Simin Nikbin. Effect of Long-term Dietary Antioxidant Supplementation on Influenza Virus Infection. *The Journals of Gerontology Series A: Biological Sciences and Medical Sciences* 55:B496-B503 (2000).

Nurk, Eha, Refsum, Helga, Drevon, Christian A., Tell, Grethe S., Nygaard, Harald A., Engedal, Knut and Smith, A. David. Intake of Flavonoid-Rich Wine, Tea, and Chocolate by Elderly Men and Women Is Associated with Better Cognitive Test Performance1–3. *Journal of Nutrition* Vol. 139, No. 1, 120-127, January 2009.

Karatzi, Kalliopi PhD, Papamichael, Christos MD, Karatzis, Emmanouil MD, Papaioannou, Theodore G. PhD, Voidonikola, Paraskevi Th.MD, Vamvakou, Giorgia, D. MD, Lekakis, John MD and Zampelas, Antonis PhD. Postprandial Improvement of Endothelial Function by Red Wine and Olive Oil Antioxidants: A Synergistic Effect of Components of the Mediterranean Diet. *Journal of the American College of Nutrition* Vol. 27, No. 4, 448-453 (2008).

Chapter 10

Anton, S.D., Morrison, C.D., Cefalu, W.T., Martin, C.K., Coulon, S., Geiselman, P., Han, H., White, C.L., Williamson, D.A. Effects of Chromium Picolinate on Food Intake and Satiety. *Diabetes Technology & Therapeutics* October 2008, Volume 10, Issue 5, Pages 405-412.

Anderson, Richard A. PhD, FACN. Chromium, Glucose Intolerance and Diabetes. *Journal of the American College of Nutrition* Vol. 17, No. 6, 548-555 (1998).

Anderson, R. A. Effects of Chromium on Body Composition and Weight Loss. *Nutrition Review* 1998 Sep, Vol 56; Number 9, pages 266-270.

Kaatsa, Gilbert R., Blumb, Kenneth, Fisherc, Jeffrey A. and Adelman, Jack A. Effects of chromium picolinate supplementation on body composition: a randomized, double-masked, placebo-controlled study. *Current Therapeutic Research* Volume 57, Issue 10, 1996, pages 747-756.

Chapter 11

Morre, DM, Kern, D, et al. Supplementation with CoQ10 lowers age-related (ar) NOX levels in healthy subjects. *Biofactors* 2008; 32(1-4): 221-30.

Gardiner, Paula, Woods, Charles and Kemper, Kathi J. Dietary supplement use among health care professionals enrolled in an online curriculum on herbs and dietary supplements. *BMC Complementary and Alternative Medicine* 2007; 7: 21.

Berman, Marius M.D., Erman, Arie Ph.D., Ben-Gal, Tuvia M.D., Dvir, Dan M.D., Georghiou, Georgios P. M.D., Stamler, Alon M.D., Vered, Yaffa Ph.D., Vidne, Bernardo A. M.D., Aravot, Dan M.D. Clinical Investigation Coenzyme Q10 in patients with end-stage heart failure awaiting cardiac transplantation: A randomized, placebo-controlled study. *Clinical Cardiol* Volume 27 Issue 5, pages 295-299.

Baggioc, E., Gandinic, R., Plancherc, A.C., Passeric, M. and Carmosino, G. Italian multicenter study on the safety and efficacy of coenzyme Q10 as adjunctive therapy in heart failure. *Molecular Aspects of Medicine* Volume 15, Supplement 1, 1994, Pages s287-s294.

Molyneux, Sarah L. PhD, Florkowski, Christopher M. MD, George, Peter M. MB, BS, Pilbrow, Anna P. PhD, Frampton, Christopher M. PhD, Lever, Michael PhD and Richards, A. Mark MD, PhD. Coenzyme Q10: An Independent Predictor of Mortality in Chronic Heart Failure. *J Am Coll Cardiol* 2008 Oct 28; 52(18), 1435-1441.

Teran, Enrique, MD, PhD. Coenzyme Q10 Supplementation and Development of Preeclampsia. *ClinicalTrials.gov* Identifier: NCT00300937.

Sena, C., Nunes, E., Gomes, A., Santos, M., Proença, T., Martins, M., Seiça, R. Supplementation of coenzyme Q10 and α-tocopherol lowers glycated hemoglobin level and lipid peroxidation in pancreas of diabetic rats. *Nutrition Research* Volume 28, Issue 2, 113-121.

Chapter 12

Columbia University. The Effect of Omega-3 Polyunsaturated Fatty Acids in Congestive Heart Failure. *ClinicalTrials.gov.* Identifier: NCT00944229.

Shah, Keyur B.; Duda, Monika K.; O'Shea, Karen M.; Sparagna, Genevieve C.; Chess, David J.; Khairallah, Ramzi J.; Robillard-Frayne, Isabelle; Xu, Wenhong; Murphy, Robert C.; Des Rosiers, Christine; Stanley, William C. The Cardioprotective Effects of Fish Oil During Pressure Overload Are Blocked by High Fat Intake. Role of Cardiac Phospholipid Remodeling. *Hypertension* 2009; 54: 605-611.

Liang, Bin, Wang, Shan, Ye, Ying-Jiang, Yang, Xiao-Dong, Wang, You-Li, Qu, Jun, Xie, Qi-Wei and Yin, Mu-Jun. Impact of postoperative omega-3 fatty acid-supplemented parenteral nutrition on clinical outcomes and immunomodulations in colorectal cancer patients. *World J Gastroenterol* 2008 April 21; 14(15): 2434-2439.

Valdivielso, Pedro, Rioja, José, García-Arias, Carlota, Sánchez-Chaparro, Miguel Angel, and González-Santos, Pedro. Omega 3 fatty acids induce a marked reduction of apolipoprotein B48 when added to fluvastatin in patients with type 2 diabetes and mixed hyperlipidemia: a preliminary report. *Cardiovascular Diabetology* 2009, 8:1.

Gonzalez-Periz, A., Horrillo,R., Ferre, N., Gronert, K., Dong, B., Moran-Salvador, Titos, E., Martinez-Clemente, E. M., Lopez-Parra, M., Arroyo, V., Claria, J. Obesity-induced insulin resistance and hepatic steatosis are alleviated by -3 fatty acids: a role for resolvins and protectins. *FASEB Journal* 2009:23: 1946-1957.

Peoples, Gregory E PhD; McLennan, Peter L PhD; Howe, Peter R C PhD; Groeller, Herbert PhD. Fish Oil Reduces Heart Rate and Oxygen Consumption During Exercise. *Journal of Cardiovascular Pharmacology* December 2008 - Volume 52 - Issue 6 - pages 540-547.

Brox, J, Bjørnstad, E, Olaussen, K, Østerud, B, Almdahl, S and Løchen, M L. Blood lipids, fatty acids, diet and lifestyle parameters in adolescents from a region in northern Norway with a high mortality from coronary heart disease. *EJCN (European Journal of Clinical Nutrition)* July 2002, Volume 56, Number 7, pages 694-700.

Donaghue Medical Research Foundation. Effects of Omega-3 Fatty Acids on Bone and Frailty. *ClinicalTrials.gov* Identifier: NCT00634686.

Logan, Alan C. Omega-3 fatty acids and major depression: A primer for the mental health professional. *Lipids in Health and Disease* 2004, 3:25.

Conklin, Dr. Sarah. Omega 3 Fatty Acids Influence Mood, Impulsivity And Personality, Study Indicates. University of Pittsburgh Medical Center (2006, March 4).

Marangell, Lauren B. M.D., Martinez, James M. M.D., Zboyan, Holly A. B.A., Kertz, Barbara M.A., Seung Kim, H. Florence M.D., and J. Puryear, Lucy M.D. A Double-Blind,

Placebo-Controlled Study of the Omega-3 Fatty Acid Docosahexaenoic Acid in the Treatment of Major Depression. *Am J Psychiatry* 160:996-998, May 2003.

S. Jazayeri, M. Tehrani-Doost; S.A. Keshavarz, M. Hosseini, A. Djazayery, H. Amini, M. Jalali, M. Peet . Comparison of therapeutic effects of omega-3 fatty acid eicosapentaenoic acid and fluoxetine, separately and in combination, in major depressive disorder. Australian and *New Zealand Journal of Psychiatry* Volume 42, Issue 3, pages 192-198.

Richardson AJ, and Puri BK. The potential role of fatty acids in attention-deficit/hyperactivity disorder. *Prostaglandins, Leukotrienes and Essential Fatty Acids* Volume 63, Issues 1-2, July 2000: pages 79-87.

Chapter 13

Clegg, D, et al. Glucosamine, Chondroitin Sulfate, and the Two in Combination for Painful Knee Osteoarthritis. *New England Journal of Medicine* 2006; 354:795-808.

Chapter 14

Kuriyama S, Shimazu T, Ohmori K, Kikuchi N, Nakaya N, Nishino Y, Tsubono Y, Tsuji I. Green tea consumption and mortality due to cardiovascular disease, cancer, and all causes in Japan: the Ohsaki study. *JAMA* 2006 Sep 13; 296(10):1255-65.

Sumpio, Bauer MD. Green Tea and the "Asian Paradox". *Journal of the American College of Surgeons* 202: 813-825 (May 2006).

Bettuzzi S, Brausi M, Rizzi F, Castagnetti G, Peracchia G, Corti A. Chemoprevention of human prostate cancer by oral administration of green tea catechins in volunteers with high-grade prostate intraepithelial neoplasia: a preliminary report from a one-year proof-of-principle study. *Cancer Res* 2006; 66(2):1234-40.

Borrelli F, Capasso R, Russo A, Ernst E. Systematic review: green tea and gastrointestinal cancer risk. *Aliment Pharmacol Ther* Mar 1, 2004;19(5):497-510.

Fukino Y, Ikeda A, Maruyama K, Aoki N, Okubo T, Iso H. Randomized controlled trial for an effect of green tea-extract powder supplementation on glucose abnormalities. *Eur J Clin Nutr* 2007 June.

Gross G, Meyer KG, Pres H, Thielert C, Tawfik H, Mescheder A. A randomized, double-blind, four-arm parallel-group, placebo-controlled Phase II/III study to investigate the clinical efficacy of two galenic formulations of Polyphenon(R) E in the treatment of external genital warts. *J Eur Acad Dermatol Venereol* 2007; 21(10):1404-12.

Hudson, Tori. Green tea enhances survival of ovarian cancer patients. *Townsend Letter for Doctors and Patients*, Dec, 2005.

Binns C, et al. Green tea consumption enhances survival of epithelial ovarian cancer patients. *Asia Pac J Clin Nutr* 2004; 12(Suppl):S116.

Imai K, Nakachi K. Cross sectional study of effects of drinking green tea on cardiovascular and liver diseases. *BMJ* 1995 Mar 18; 310(6981):693-6.

Zhang XG, Xu P, Liu Q, Yu CH, Zhang Y, Chen SH, Li YM. Effect of tea polyphenol on cytokine gene expression in rats with alcoholic liver disease. *Hepatobiliary Pancreat Dis Int* 2006 May; 5(2):268-72.

Wang, H, Wen Y, Yan X, Guo, H, Rycroft, JA, Boon N, Kovacs, EM, Mela, DJ. Effects of catechin enriched green tea on body composition. *Obesity* (Silver Spring) 2009 Aug 13.

Boon, Niels Dr. Green Tea Promotes Weight Loss, New Research Finds. *Medical News Today*. 10 Sep 2009.

Maki, Kevin C., Reeves, Matthew S., Farmer, Mildred, Yasunaga, Koichi, Matsuo, Noboru, Katsuragi, Yoshihisa, Komikado, Masanori, Tokimitsu, Ichiro, Wilder, Donna, Jones, Franz, Blumberg, Jeffrey B. and Cartwright, Yolanda. Green Tea Catechin Consumption Enhances Exercise-Induced Abdominal Fat Loss in Overweight and Obese Adults. *Journal of Nutrition* Vol. 139, No. 2, 264-270, February 2009.

Rueff, José, Gaspar, Jorge and Laires, António. Structural requirements for mutagenicity of flavonoids upon nitrosation. A structure—activity study. *Mutagenesis* vol. 10 no. 4 pp. 325-328, 1995.

Chapter 15

Rabbani, Ramin and Topol, Eric J. Strategies to achieve coronary arterial plaque stabilization. *Cardiovascular Research* 1999 41(2):402-417.

Sumner, M., Elliott-Eller, M., Weidner, G., Daubenmier, J., Chew, M., Marlin, R., Raisin, C., Ornish, D. Effects of Pomegranate Juice Consumption on Myocardial Perfusion in Patients with Coronary Heart Disease. *The American Journal of Cardiology* Volume 96, Issue 6, Pages 810-814.

Ignarro, LJ, Byrns, Re, Sumi, D, de Nigris, F, Napoli, C. Pomegranate juice protects nitric oxide against oxidative destruction and enhances the biological actions of nitric oxide. *Nitric Oxide* 2006 Sep; 15(2): 93-102.

Chapter 16

Fish, E., Beverstein, G., Olson, D., Reinhardt, S., Garren, M., Gould, J. QS82. Vitamin D Status of Morbidly Obese Bariatric Surgery Patients. *Journal of Surgical Research* Volume 144, Issue 2, Pages 301-301.

Holick, Michael F. M.D., Ph.D. Vitamin D Deficiency. *N Engl J Med* 2007; 357: 266-81.

Lipworth, L., Rossi, M., McLaughlin, J. K., Negri, E., Talamini, R., Levi, F., Franceschi, S. and La Vecchia, C. Dietary vitamin D and cancers of the oral cavity and esophagus. *Annals of Oncology* 2009 20(9):1576-1581.

Chlebowski, Rowan T., Johnson, Karen C., Kooperberg, Charles, Pettinger, Mary, Wactawski-Wende, Jean, Rohan, Tom, Rossouw, Jacques, Lane, Dorothy, O'Sullivan, Mary Jo , Yasmeen, Shagufta, Hiatt, Robert A., Shikany, James M., Vitolins, Mara, Khandekar, Janu, Hubbell, F. Allan for the Women's Health. Calcium Plus Vitamin D Supplementation and the Risk of Breast Cancer. *JNCI Journal of the National Cancer Institute* 2008; 100(22): 1581-1591.

Prepared by the editors at Harvard Health Publications in consultation with Meir J. Stampfer, M.D., Dr.P.H., Professor of Epidemiology and Nutrition, Harvard School of Public Health. *Vitamins and Minerals: What you need to know, a Special Health Report from Harvard Medical School,* Copyright © 2008 by Harvard University.

Theodoratou, E, Farrington, SM, Tenesa, A, McNeill, G, Cetnarskyj, R, Barnetson, RA, Porteous, ME, Dunlop, MG, Campbell, H. Modification of the inverse association between dietary vitamin D intake and colorectal cancer risk by a FokI variant supports a chemoprotective action of Vitamin D intake mediated through VDR binding. *Int J Cancer* 2008; 123(9):2170-9.

American Heart Association (2009, March 18). Low Vitamin D Levels Associated With Several Risk Factors In Teenagers. *Science Daily.*

Reis, JP, von Muhlen, D, Miller, III ER, et al. Vitamin D status and cardiovascular disease risk factors in the us adolescent population. *AHA 49th Annual Conference on Cardiovascular Disease Epidemiology and Prevention;* March 11, 2009; Palm Harbor, FL. Poster P54.

Saintonge, S, Bang, H, Vogiatzi, MG, et al. Is the relevance of vitamin D deficiency increasing? Data from the National Health and Nutrition Examination Survey: 1988-1994 and 2001-2006. *AHA 49th Annual Conference on Cardiovascular Disease Epidemiology and Prevention;* March 11, 2009; Palm Harbor, FL. Abstract 9.

Medical College of Georgia. Vitamin D Supplement Study for Adolescents (VIP). *ClinicalTrials.gov* Identifier: NCT00909454.

Hilliard, Jennifer. Not enough vitamin D in the diet could mean too much fat on adolescents. *Medical College of Georgia News.* - 2009 March 12

The Peninsula College of Medicine and Dentistry(2009, January 24). Low Levels Of Vitamin D Link To Cognitive Problems In Older People. *Science Daily.*

Breijawi, N., Eckardt, A., Pitton, M.B., Hoelzl, A.J., Giesa, M., von Stechow, D., Haid, F., Drees, P. Bone Mineral Density and Vitamin D Status in Female and Male Patients with Osteoarthritis of the Knee or Hip. *European Surgical Research* 2009; 42(1): 1-10.

Merlino LA, Curtis J, Mikuls TR, Cerhan JR, Criswell LA, Saag KG; Iowa Women's Health Study. Vitamin D intake is inversely associated with rheumatoid arthritis: results from the Iowa Women's Health Study. *Arthritis Rheum* 2006 Nov; 54(11):3719-20.

The University of Colorado Denver School of Medicine. Vitamin D deficiency may increase risk of colds, flu. Published: Monday, February 23, 2009 - 17:11 in *Health & Medicine*.

Melamed, Michal L., MD, MHS, Michos, Erin D. MD, Post, Wendy MD, MS and Astor, Brad PhD. 25-hydroxyl Vitamin D Levels and the Risk of Mortality in the General Population. *Arch Intern Med* 2008 August 11; 168(15): 1629–1637.

Kubzansky, LD, Berkman, LF, Glass, TA and Seeman, TE. Is educational attainment associated with shared determinants of health in the elderly? Findings from the MacArthur Studies of Successful Aging. *Psychosomatic Medicine* Vol 60, Issue 5 578-585.

Diets That Reduce Calories Lead to Weight Loss, Regardless of Carbohydrate, Protein or Fat Content. Long-Term Study Shows That Attending Counselling Sessions Also Key to Promoting Weight Loss. *Harvard School of Public Health 2009* Releases Wednesday, February 25, 2009.

Acknowledgements

It takes many supportive people to give life to a concept and a book like *Health Is Wealth*. To each and every person who has been a part of the development of this book; we would like to offer a humble and heartfelt, "Thank you!"

Thank you as well, to the readers of this book who believe that *"healthcare is really self care"* and who are willing to help share our wellness message with their families, friends, and co-workers. We wrote *Health Is Wealth* for the purpose of empowering our readers to take charge of their own wellness and make a positive and lasting impact on their quality of life.

Our deepest thanks to:

Our families and friends for their constant love and support throughout the book development process.

Our friend and business partner, Dave Brubaker, whose entrepreneurial spirit and business acumen help guide our success.

Our book production team: Maryanna Young, Personal Value Coaching for her friendship, leadership and project management; Shannon Tracy for her research support; Amy Meyer for her constant support and extra effort "down the stretch;" Kelly Antonczak for her attention to detail; Brook Dryden for financial management; Cari Campbell and Fuel3 Advertising for cover design; Tim Vandehey for his tremendous patience and story-telling skills; Nick and Betsy Zelinger and NZ Graphics for interior design and editing; Lloyd Jassin for legal advice and direction; Peggy Jordan and the Working Words Copywriting team for proofreading and attention to detail; and Stephen Watts, Denny Hooten, Jay Brubaker, Don Brown, Joel Margulies and Margaret McGinnis for helping us shape our message.

We would also like to offer special thanks to the global Herbalife family, Herbalife's Chief Executive Michael O. Johnson and his outstanding Executive Team, and our colleagues on the Herbalife Scientific Advisory Board, Dr. David Heber, Dr. Steve Henig and Dr. Luigi Gratton for their support of our *Health Is Wealth* message.

SPREAD THE WELLNESS!

Health Is Wealth books are available at quantity discounts for orders of 10 or more copies. Additional volume discounts apply for quantities of 100, 500 or 1000.

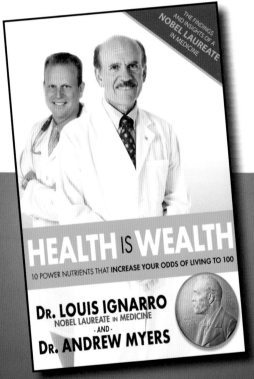

ISBN 978-0-9790229-1-3
Retail Price $18.95 US | $21.95 CAN

To find out about our discounts for orders of 10 or more copies for individuals, corporations, academic use, associations and organizations, please call us at (800) 817-0018.

To find out about our discount program for resellers, please contact our Special Sales department at ameyer@nutragenetics.net

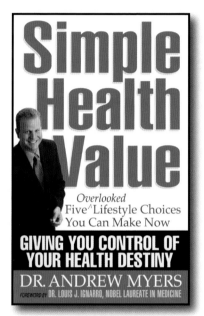
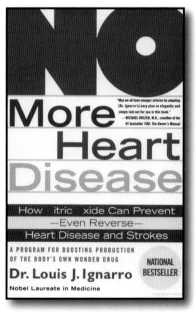

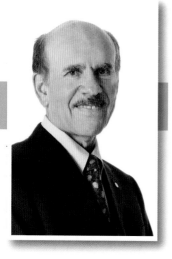

DR. IGNARRO was awarded the Nobel Prize in Medicine in 1998 for his discoveries surrounding Nitric Oxide. Dr. Ignarro's research into Nitric Oxide and cardiovascular health has been called "one of the greatest discoveries in human health." Dr. Ignarro is a Research Pharmacologist and distinguished Professor of Pharmacology at the UCLA School of Medicine. Dr. Ignarro is the author of the best-selling book, **NO More Heart Disease.**

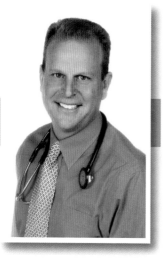

DR. MYERS is a naturopathic physician who specialized in nutrition and preventative health. Dr Myers has nearly 20 years experience in the field of natural medicine – including patient care, clinical research, professional speaking and product development. Dr Myers is the President and Chief Science Officer of NutraGenetics, a global product development company founded by Nobel Laureate Dr. Louis Ignarro and is also the author of **Simple Health Value.**